Toxic Immune Syndrome Cookbook

Yeast-Free
Hypo-Allergenic
Recipes to
Support Your
Immune System

**Comprehensive
Health Centers**

W.R. Kellas, Ph.D.

Published by:
Comprehensive Health Centers
4403 Manchester Avenue, Suite 206
Encinitas CA 92024
619-632-9042

Design, layout and editing by Andrea Sharon Dworkin
Illustration by CorelDraw Clipart, © Corel Corporation 1994

Publisher's cataloging information:

Kellas, W.R.
   Toxic immune system cookbook; yeast-free hypo-allergenic
recipes to support your immune system. 2d ed.
           p.   cm.
       1. Immunologic diseases-diet therapy-recipes. 2. Alternative medicine.
3. Diet. 4. Cookery. I. Title

RM219   641.563   ISBN 0-9636491-0-8

Printed in United States of America

TABLE OF CONTENTS

Introduction

This book was compiled for the benefit of those people, possibly including yourself, who suffer from immune system related health problems. How do these health problems come about? Toxins and chemicals that most of us are exposed to set up conditions that favor the growth of yeast and other microorganisms. Both the primary toxic suppressors (chemicals, metals, electromagnetic radiation) and the secondary suppressors (yeast and microorganisms) can cause the immune system to appear to malfunction as it copes with the invaders as best it can. Many health problems and symptoms can result, including allergies, frequent infections, and fatigue.

The recipes in this book help boost the immune system in several ways:

- Foods which provide optimal nutrition to support the body are used as ingredients.

- Relatively pure foods are used to minimize exposure to toxic food additives.

- Foods such as sugars, simple carbohydrates, fermented products and fruit which feed yeast and fungus are eliminated or minimized.

- Foods which are most likely to be allergenic, such as dairy, wheat, corn, and soy are eliminated or minimized.

This book came about from the experience of Dr. Bill Kellas. He developed the crippling autoimmune disease ankylosing spondylitis in the early 1970s. After years of research and self-experimentation, he found that a regimen which works with the body, including dietary modifications, keeps his illness under control. He then started working with people who had a wide variety of chronic and immune-related illnesses using some of the same methods.

Bill's wife Laurie developed many of these recipes for him over the years, incorporating those foods which benefit the most and harm the least. Now these recipes are available to you.

Bon Appetit! We wish you success in your journey toward optimal health.

Information For Getting The Best Use Out Of This Cookbook

This section describes the basic philosophy of this cookbook. Once you understand what foods you should and shouldn't eat and why, you can make the best food choices for yourself. The recipes in this cookbook incorporate those ingredients most conducive to immune system health.

Not all bodies are created equal, of course. If your doctor or your own body's sensitivities or reactions tell you not to eat a certain food, then follow the advice of your body or doctor rather than this or any book.

In many cases the use of this cookbook will follow the 8-day detoxification diet utilized by Comprehensive Health Centers - Medical Center. This diet involves the use of foods with very low yeast-feeding or allergenic potential to clean out the body and starve yeast and other microorganisms. In addition, the person's reaction to the diet can provide important diagnostic clues.

Once your system is cleared of most or all possible allergens and yeast feeders, it should be relatively easy to monitor your reactions to individual foods as they are added. This monitoring can take the form of watching for a return of your symptoms such as fatigue, irritability, or headache. Another way to see how your body is tolerating foods is to check the pH of your urine every morning. More information on this testing technique is given in the back of the book. The recipes in this cookbook are ideal for the purpose of monitoring reactivity, as they are relatively simple and use foods that are reasonably pure and additive-free.

As you get healthier, you may find that foods that used to cause you trouble can now be eaten in moderation.

Some of the ingredients included in some of the recipes are less than optimal because they have slightly greater allergenic or yeast-feeding potential. Not everyone who is using this cookbook has the same problems or to the same degree, so recipes with these ingredients are included. The optimal and less-than-optimal grains, vegetables, etc. are listed and discussed in this section so you (and your doctor) can make your own decisions about whether to include them. Similarly, some recipes have frying in oil as a tastier but less healthful option.

Rotate your foods

To avoid or minimize allergic reactions, rotate your grains and proteins every five days. It takes at least 72 hours to clear allergens from your body, and so eating a particular food only one day out of five will lessen the chance of allergic reactions. It is often possible to eat foods to which one is mildly sensitive without reaction if the foods are rotated. An example of food rotation:

> Day 1 - Salmon/Millet
> Day 2 - Chicken/Quinoa
> Day 3 - Tuna/Amaranth
> Day 4 - Turkey/Brown Rice
> Day 5 - Mackerel/Buckwheat

Then repeat and rotate in gluten grains (oats, barley, rye) on every fifth day and see how you feel. Watch out for fatigue, mucus (runny or stuffy nose), rashes, aches, gas, headaches or other symptoms.

Diet composition

Ideally, your diet should con-
sist of:

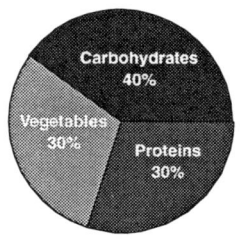

- 30% protein
- 40% grains
- 30% vegetables

Oils are also crucial for optimal nutrition, as discussed later in
this section. Oil is a component of most protein sources and is
also added to some of the recipes.

Use organically grown foods whenever possible.

Protein

The best sources of protein are:

- Chicken and turkey
- Lamb
- Fish
- Eggs

If a land animal is larger than you, its protein is harder to digest
and will probably cause allergies. You should use it to pull a
plow, not as food.

Cold-water fish is generally the healthiest, then warm-water
fish. Ground-crawling fish such as catfish are usually the least
healthful.

Always take skin and fat off chicken. Save chicken and turkey
bones all week to make broth on weekend. (Store in the freezer
until needed.)

Chicken, turkey, lamb, and even fish in some cases can be used interchangeably in most recipes.

Eggs should be cooked soft-boiled or poached. Hard-cooked eggs can be used only without the yolks, as hard-cooked egg yolk is a concentrated source of cholesterol which can burden the liver. When using raw eggs, hold the whole egg under hot water for one minute. The heat inactivates the enzyme avidin which would otherwise destroy the nutrient biotin.

Other sources of protein, which are not as complete and should be combined with complex carbohydrates, include:

- Beans, lentils, legumes, dried peas
- Nuts, except peanuts and pistachios which can contain toxic mold
- Seeds such as sunflower seeds, sesame seeds

These protein sources also contain carbohydrates, a factor to take into consideration when combining nearly equal parts protein and carbohydrate.

To cook kidney beans: Boil in water for 10 minutes. Drain water. Boil again in new water for 10 more minutes. Drain again. Refill with new water, boil again for 10 minutes. Drain again. Refill with water and cook until beans are soft (approximately 45 minutes). The use of enzymes or a product called Beano may reduce gas or discomfort associated with eating beans.

Complex Carbohydrates / Grains

Grains should be eaten in their most basic unrefined form possible; for example, brown rice rather than white, and whole grains rather than flour. However, if you are allergic to brown rice, white rice may not cause a problem, and whole wheat flour may work better than whole grain wheat for someone with a wheat allergy.

Fermentation: Grains should be cooked until crunchy/chewy, not soggy. If grains are overcooked, the outside shells crack and nutrients are lost. In addition, overcooked grains are more subject to fermentation. Cook only enough for the current meal and either discard or immediately freeze any leftovers. Even properly cooked grains can ferment if left sitting on the stove or more slowly in the refrigerator.

Further understanding of the fermentation issue can be provided by the following chart, explained on the following page:

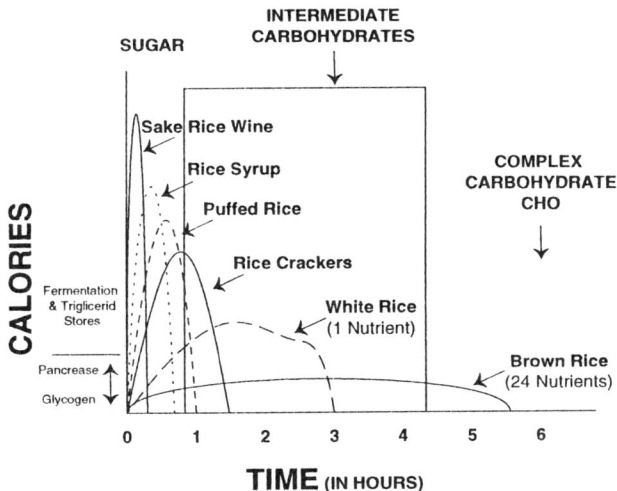

Fermentation of grains, which can occur when grains are over-cooked or allowed to sit after cooking, causes grains to turn into what the food processing industry turns them into: sugar and syrup, vinegar, and alcohol. Wine, syrup, and vinegar release sugars into the bloodstream more rapidly than do brown rice or other complex carbohydrates. This rapid rise in sugar can feed yeast and other microorganisms in a way that the complex carbohydrates do not.

In addition, a too-rapid rise in blood sugar levels can cause an increase in the secretion of insulin, a hormone which helps to moderate the level of sugar in the blood. This insulin release can lead to food cravings and to the production of triglycerides, which can cause fat to be stored in the body.

Use of the grains: Most recipes can be done with any of the grains interchangeably.

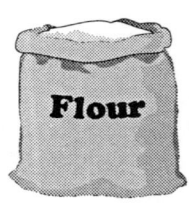

When recipes call for flour, use rice, millet, oat, buckwheat, barley or rye flour. Do not use wheat flour. If gluten sensitive, try one type of flour at a time starting with rice flour. Ideally, flour should be fresh ground when needed to avoid loss of nutrients. Barley flour is most similar to wheat flour.

Recommended grains: These have little or no gluten, a protein to which some people may be sensitive, and are less allergenic than other grains:
- Brown rice
- Amaranth
- Millet
- Buckwheat groats
- Quinoa
- Teff

The following grains are also healthy, but they contain gluten:
- Barley
- Rye
- Triticale
- Oat groats
- Kamut
- Spelt

Kamut and spelt are related to wheat, but are less likely than wheat to cause problems. If you are allergic to wheat, use these with caution. When rotating foods, consider wheat, kamut, and spelt to be in the same category - if you use one of these, do not use any of these (wheat, kamut, or spelt) for another five days. Be aware that bulghur and cous cous are forms of wheat.

The following are nutritious but contain both wheat and gluten, both common allergens:
- Bulghur wheat
- Cous cous

To prepare grains:

Rinse grains in cold water only if they seem gritty, since grains contain B vitamins which are readily washed away. Quinoa should be rinsed at least twice as it has a bitter tasting coating.

Bring liquid (water or stock) to a full boil. Add Real Salt or mineral salt if desired.

Add the grain to the boiling liquid and stir once.

Cover pot. Reduce heat to the lowest setting and cook until all the liquid is absorbed. (See time table on next page)

Use the taste test to determine if the grains are done. They should still be a little crunchy. Cooking times given below are approximate, and may differ with altitude.

GRAIN MEASUREMENT CHART

GRAIN 1 cup	LIQUID (cups)	COOKING TIME	YIELDS (cups)
Amaranth	1	7 min.	3
Barley	2	30 min.	3
Brown Rice	1 1/2	25 min.	2
Buckwheat Groats	2	5 min.	2
Bulghur Wheat	1	15 min.	2
Cous cous	1	3 min.	2
Millet	1	7 min.	2
Oat Groats	2	25 min.	3
Quinoa	1	7 min.	2
Rye	2	30 min.	3
Teff	1	7 min.	2
Triticale	2	15 min.	3
Spelt	1	12 min.	1 1/2
Kamut	1	17 min.	2

Oils

Healthy oils are needed for optimal body function. Unhealthy oils are treated by the body as a toxic waste product. Healthy oils can be made unhealthy if handled improperly.

Healthy oils fall into three categories based on their chemical structure, their sources, and the way they are used in the body:

- Omega I   - olive oil
- Omega III   - salmon, mackerel, cold water fish, flax-seed, canola oils
- Omega VI   - sesame, safflower, sunflower oils

These oils should be bought fresh and used cold or added to foods after cooking. The three enemies of oils are **heat, air,** and **light**. Heating oils or frying with them, keeping them for long periods of time, or exposing them to light for lengthy periods can change their chemical structure to an unhealthy form. It is best to cook in water or broth, then add oil. Any fats which are solid or semi-solid (fully or partially saturated or hydrogenated), such as margarine or lard, are generally harmful.

An easy-to-digest oil recipe which contains all three types of oil is:

      1 cup olive oil
      1/4 cup sesame, safflower, or sunflower oil
      1/3 cup flaxseed or canola oil
      1 1/2 cups water
      1/4 bottle E Gem vitamin E oil drops (or 1200
         IU vitamin E oil)
      1/8 cup liquid lecithin

Coat blender with sesame oil. Add lecithin to bottom as first ingredient. Put all ingredients in a blender and mix thoroughly. You can add different permitted seasonings to change the flavor - try garlic, dry mustard, lemon juice, and/or Italian seasoning. You may want to over-season as oil absorbs flavors. Keep refrigerated at all times. Put on grains or vegetables - about 1-4 T. Keeps about one week.

Vegetables

Vegetables should comprise about 30% of your diet. Only non-sweet vegetables should be used. They should be eaten raw, steamed, or steam-fried ("fried" in water or broth instead of oil). If cooked, vegetables should be still somewhat crunchy rather than overcooked to preserve nutrients and avoid fermentation. More cooking suggestions are in the Vegetables section of this cookbook.

Any vegetable that tastes sweet is probably too sweet to eat. Sweet foods feed yeast, bacteria, and fungus.

Recommended vegetables:

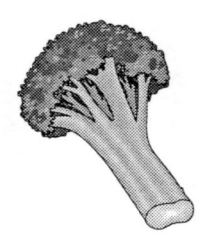
Almost any green vegetables *except* peas, lima beans, and bell peppers
Cauliflower, cabbage, broccoli
Summer squash such as yellow squash or zucchini. Summer squash has thin edible skins.
Onions, garlic

Not recommended - too sweet or too high in carbohydrates - can ferment
> Peas
> Winter squash such as butternut or banana squash has non-edible skins and sweet taste
> Carrots (although one raw carrot a day is permissible)
> Tomatoes
> Beets
> Sweet red peppers, bell peppers
> Sweet potatoes, yams
> Corn

Potatoes
Lima beans
Fruit

Not recommended - high allergenic potential
Corn
Tomatoes
Fruit

Not recommended - other
Mushrooms are a form of fungus (related to mold) and
are conducive to fungus growth and allergy
Canned vegetables
Pickled or preserved vegetables often contain vinegar,
colors, and/or preservatives

Should be avoided by people with a tendency to arthritis (night-shade vegetables)
Green (Bell) or red peppers
Tomatoes
Eggplant

Dairy

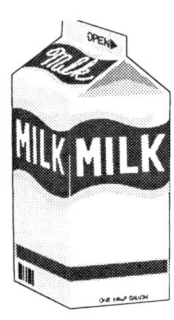

Dairy products are generally allergenic, as milk is made for a calf which has four stomachs to digest it and the proteins are too complex for us to break down easily. For this reason these recipes have no dairy products (milk or cheese) except for two: yogurt and butter. Butter is almost 100% fat with little or no milk protein, although it is less healthful than oil.

13

Yogurt contains both enzymes and lactobacillus (beneficial bacteria) to help in its digestion. However, it is important to use only good quality yogurt such as Alta Dena brand without flavors or sweetening. Many commercial brands of yogurt have been pasteurized, which kills both enzymes and lactobacillus. Cooking with yogurt is not recommended, as the heat would have the same detrimental effect.

Problems with dairy products - gastrointestinal pain or gas - can be due to either milk allergy or lactose intolerance. If you are allergic to the casein protein in milk, then you will likely also have trouble with yogurt. However, if your problem is with lactose intolerance, then you may be able to handle a good quality yogurt without difficulty since the yogurt contains the enzymes which help with digestion that you may be lacking.

Plain yogurt can be substituted for or mixed with mayonnaise. Some people may be able to tolerate small amounts - two ounces or less.

If you are unable to tolerate yogurt, homemade mayonnaise or an oil and butter mixture may be substituted in some recipes.

Dairy products, like meat, are high in arachidonic acid, which increases the amount of the prostaglandin PGE2, which promotes inflammation. If you have a tendency to inflammatory conditions such as menstrual cramps, cancer, or arthritis, it may be wise to avoid or limit all meat and dairy products, including butter and yogurt.

People who are sensitive to cow's milk products may be able to tolerate goat's milk or nut milks such as almond milk.

Other Recommended Foods

Recommended teas:
>Spearmint Tea
>Desert Herb Tea
>Red Raspberry Herb Tea

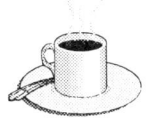

Recommended seasonings:
>Celery Salt, Sea Salt, Celery Seed, Dill Weed,
>Marjoram, Mrs. Dash, Dry Mustard, Cayenne,
>Garlic Powder, Onion Powder, Cinnamon

Other Foods Not Permitted or Not Recommended

These feed yeast or set up a fermenting environment:
>Sweets - sugar, honey, syrup, corn syrup
>Fruit, especially dried, and fruit juice, although lemon
>>and lemon juice are permitted
>Breads
>Alcohol - Beer is the worst, then wine, then hard alco-
>>hol. As an alternative have Bitters over ice
>Vinegar, also found in most mayonnaise, salad dressing,
>>ketchup, prepared mustard
>Carbonated drinks, including carbonated water, make
>>the blood more alkaline, a condition favored by yeast
>>and other microorganisms.

These are toxic:
>Saccharin, Nutri-Sweet, any artificial sweetener
>Fried foods
>Margarine
>Caffeine
>Alcohol

Water

Use only bottled or filtered water, not tap water, for cooking or drinking.

Cookware To Use

Recommended:
- Visions glass pots and pans
- Corningware
- Pyrex

Not Recommended:
- Stainless steel
- Iron
- Aluminum
- Copper
- Teflon or Silverstone

Basic Rules and Helpful Hints and Suggestions

- If it tastes sweet it probably is and will therefore ferment.

- If a food causes gas, it is fermenting or you are allergic to it and the food should be either reduced or eliminated. Enzymes taken orally may help with digestion. If so, use them; if not, the problem may be allergy or fermentation rather than digestion. Lactase is a good enzyme for digesting milk, and protease can help with beans or meat.

- Sea salt, Real Salt, Celtic salt, mineral salt, or celery salt can be added to recipes, if desired. (Regular table salt contains sugar and aluminum chlorohydrate - read labels even on health food store brands)

- Use arrowroot as a thickener: 1 T. arrowroot (more or less) to 1 cup liquid. Heat until thickened. Add more liquid if too thick or more arrowroot if too thin.

- Cooking half as hot, twice as long preserves natural enzymes.

- Mayonnaise - only use homemade recipe in this cookbook. All store-bought mayonnaise contains vinegar.

- Remember, the key to good tasting meals are sauces, dressings, herbs and seasonings.

- Regarding our eating habits and good health - we discipline ourselves to do the things we don't want to do so we can have the things we want to have.

Eating Out

Eating out is always a challenge to those most concerned with maintaining total health.

We have found that fast food restaurants are the most difficult. They are quick and almost too easy - leading to temptations. If you must, choose one that has a salad bar. Remember to combine foods in a 30/30/40 ratio as discussed.

Breakfast from a restaurant could include oatmeal and/or poached eggs. Not much else is safe for many patients to eat.

Lunches and dinners are more easily adjustable to this program. Many restaurants today accommodate a more healthful diet. Choose restaurants that have salad bars or steamed vegetable platters, grilled fish or poultry. Take your own salad dressing in a small container.

Always ask how food is prepared; no one should object. Ask for sauces or salad dressings to be left off or placed on the side, for butter instead of margarine, and for lemon slices on your plate. Always be courteous.

If you follow these simple guidelines you can enjoy eating out with very little inconvenience and without sacrificing your health.

Take a night off!

Abbreviations used in recipes:
    T = tablespoon   t = teaspoon

A Sample Week's Menus
* indicates recipe found in this cookbook

Monday (chicken / millet)
Breakfast
    Millet muffins*
    Sliced chicken breast
Lunch
    Veggie-potato salad*
    Add chicken chunks to salad
Dinner
    Baked chicken breast supreme*
    Broccoli
    Grain pilaf* (use millet)

Tuesday (salmon and lamb / oats)
Breakfast
    Grain and vegetable breakfast* (use oats)
Lunch
    Salmon patties with poached egg*
    Tossed green salad* with
    Olive oil dressing*
Dinner
    Plain lentil soup*
    Lamb chops
    Yellow summer squash and yogurt*

Wednesday (turkey / rice)
Breakfast
    Easy breakfast sausage*
    Rice cakes*
Lunch
    Rice and cabbage* (with turkey)
    Dilled cucumber salad*

19

Dinner
> Turkey meatloaf*
> Broccoli
> Rice pilaf*

Thursday (tuna / buckwheat)
Breakfast
> Roasted grain breakfast cereal* (use buckwheat)
Lunch
> Tuna salad with cut-up raw vegetables and...
> Mayonnaise*
Dinner
> Baked fish with spinach* (use fresh tuna)
> Fattoush salad*
> Toasted buckwheat with butter and seasonings

Friday (chicken / quinoa)
Breakfast
> Grain and vegetable breakfast* (use quinoa)
Lunch
> Chicken broth* with
> Egg dumplings*
> Quinoa - Vidalia salad
Dinner
> Confetti casserole* (use quinoa instead of rice)
> Tossed green salad* with
> Curried mayonnaise dressing*

Saturday (fish / millet and barley)
Breakfast
>   Whole grain yogurt pancakes* (use millet flour)
>   Poached eggs
Lunch
>   Mock lobster*
>   Grain pilaf* (use barley)

Dinner
>   Spinach surprise dip* with raw vegetables
>   Skewered shrimp and vegetables*
>   Millet croquettes*

Sunday (turkey / rice)
Breakfast
>   Italian sausage*
>   Whole grain yogurt waffles*
Lunch
>   Egg drop and sprout soup*
>   Fried rice* (use turkey)
Dinner
>   Thanksgiving turkey*
>   Turkey stuffing*
>   Tossed green salad* with
>   Olive oil dressing*
>   Spinach

BREAKFAST

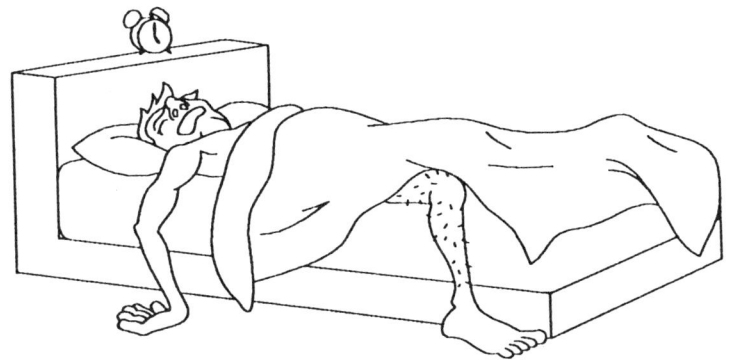

EASY BREAKFAST SAUSAGE

1 lb. ground turkey
1/4 to 1 t. sage
1/4 to 1/2 t. marjoram (optional)
1/4 to 1/2 t. thyme (optional)
1/4 to 1/2 t. coriander (optional)
1/2 t. sea salt
1/8 t. pepper
1 to 3 T. water

or

ITALIAN SAUSAGE

1 lb. ground turkey
1 medium onion, minced
1 t. sea salt
1 garlic clove, minced
1 bay leaf, finely crumbled
1/2 t. pepper
1/2 t. fennel seed, crushed
1/4 t. paprika
1/8 t. thyme
1/8 t. cayenne pepper

Sausage casings are available from your butcher. Refrigerated they will keep for 2 years. If using casings, soak in water for 2 hours or overnight in the refrigerator.

Choose the sausage you want to make. Sprinkle the seasonings over the ground meat. Knead until thoroughly blended. Make into patties, a meatloaf or stuff into sausage casings by hand or with a sausage horn. Make a large roll or tie off in 5" to 18" links with string. Refrigerate in airtight containers for 2 to 3

(continued on next page)

days to allow flavors to blend. If you plan to use the sausage immediately the spices will not be as strong.

Cooking Instructions:

Patties: Bake at 350 degrees for 40 minutes or until golden brown.

Loaf: Set loaf pan in another pan of hot water in oven. Bake at 350 degrees for 1 1/2 hours or until meat thermometer reaches 160 degrees.

Roll or links: Cover with water in skillet. Simmer for 20-30 minutes. Drain water and cook until light brown.

Note: Sheldon's chicken and turkey dogs, available at health food stores, are a healthful alternative to homemade sausage.

OAT GRIDDLE CAKES

3/4 c. cooked oatmeal
1 1/4 to 1 1/2 cups water
1 egg
2 T. oil
3/4 cup oat flour
1 t. baking powder
1/4 t. cinnamon

Mix all ingredients together and spoon onto non-stick skillet or one covered with a thin layer of olive oil. Spread mixture in pan to make a flat round pancake, about 3" in diameter. Cook like regular pancakes.

STEAMED EGGS WITH SALMON

1/2 cup plus 2 T. water
5 large eggs
dash of pepper
1 can (7 3/4 oz.) salmon, drained and flaked
1 T. green onion, minced

In a 10-inch skillet bring water to a boil over moderately high heat. Beat eggs in a bowl with pepper and pour eggs into skillet. Reduce heat. Cook about 2 minutes, stirring constantly with a large spoon or pancake turner and scraping large pieces of set egg from bottom of skillet. When almost all liquid is gone, stir in salmon and green onions. Continue stirring and cook a few seconds longer, until all liquid is absorbed. Serve immediately. Serves 4.

MILLET MUFFINS

1 cup raw millet
2 cups water
1/4 cup olive oil
1 T. butter
2 eggs
1/2 cup oat flour

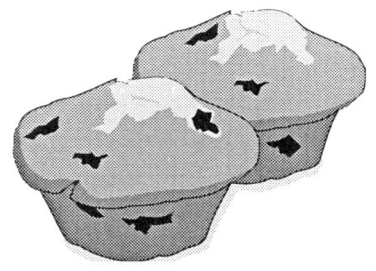

Cook raw millet in water for 15 minutes, stirring occasionally, until all water is absorbed. Remove from heat. Stir in butter until melted. Add remaining ingredients. Mix well. Put in lightly greased muffin tins, or muffin cups, and bake at 325 degrees for 30 minutes.

STEEL-CUT OATMEAL

Oatmeal can be prepared in a variety of ways, and they're all good. This recipe uses long, slow cooking and steel-cut oats (each individual oat cut into about 3 pieces by blade-fitted steel rollers) to get a delightfully creamy-style oatmeal.

2/3 cup steel-cut oats
1 cup boiling water
cinnamon
ground nutmeg
1 pat butter

Add oats to boiling water, cover and simmer 10-15 minutes over very low heat. Top with cinnamon and nutmeg.. Serve with a pat of butter.

RICE CAKES

1 egg, well beaten
1/4 cup water, and enough plain yogurt to make 1/3 cup of liquid. Mix well.
2 t. grated onion
2 cups cooked rice
1/4 cup rice flour
1 1/2 t. baking powder

Combine egg with liquid and onion. Stir in rice. Combine rice flour and baking powder and add to rice mixture, mixing slightly. Drop by tablespoon onto hot griddle. Cook until brown, then turn and flatten slightly, and brown second side. Makes 10 to 12 cakes.

WHOLE GRAIN YOGURT PANCAKES

1 cup plain, whole yogurt
1 cup water
1 to 3 eggs
1 t. baking powder
2 cups flour: rye, oat, millet or buckwheat
1/4 cup (or less) oil (optional)

In large bowl place yogurt, water, eggs, baking powder and oil. Mix well. Add flour, beating only until large lumps disappear. Batter may also be mixed in the blender. Cook on a skillet or griddle lightly greased with olive oil over medium-high heat (375 degrees). Freeze extras and heat in toaster for snacks or busy mornings.

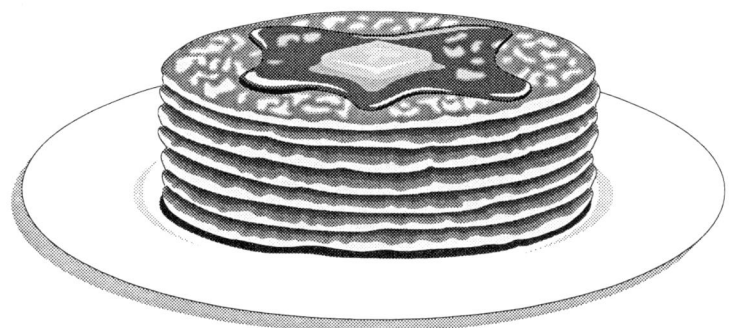

ROASTED GRAIN BREAKFAST CREAM CEREAL

1 to 1 1/2 cups grains (rice, millet, rye, barley, oats, buckwheat,
   spelt, or kamut)
4 cups water

Topping: butter, cinnamon

Wash and clean whole grains, if necessary. Drain and dry.
Roast grains in a 300 degree oven until lightly browned, using a
large baking pan. Blend or process roasted grains until as fine
as flour - a coffee grinder can be used. Bring water to a boil.
Slowly sprinkle in one cup of blended grain flour, stirring constantly until well mixed. Reduce heat, if necessary, to prevent
boiling over. Continue cooking and stirring for 20 to 25 minutes, until water is absorbed. Top with cinnamon and a pat of
butter. Store remaining grain flour, preferably in freezer, for future use. Makes 4 servings.

SWEET RICE

1 cup cooked brown rice
1/4 t. cinnamon
dash of nutmeg
dash of allspice

Stir spices into hot rice and serve. Top with butter (optional).

WHOLE GRAIN YOGURT WAFFLES

2 to 4 eggs, separated
1/2 cup yogurt
1 cup water
1/4 to 1/2 cup olive oil
1/2 t. baking powder
2 cups flour

Beat egg whites until stiff. Set aside. In a large bowl beat yolks with yogurt. Add remaining ingredients, beating after each addition. Fold in beaten egg whites. Pour into a pre-heated waffle iron that is lightly greased with olive oil and cook until it stops steaming.

Flavor choices: Add any of these to waffle mixture:

1/2 t. ground cinnamon
1/4 t. ground ginger
1/8 t. ground mace
1/2 t. ground cloves
1/2 t. ground nutmeg
1/2 t. allspice

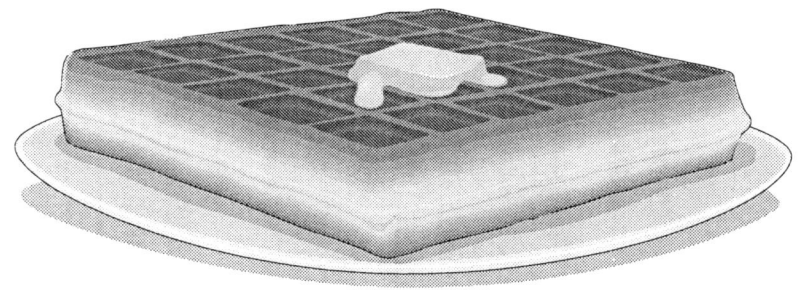

RICE PANCAKES

Follow the Yogurt Pancake recipe using 4 eggs, separated. Beat the egg whites until stiff with a pinch of cream of tartar. Use 2 cups brown rice flour and 2 T. melted butter. After mixing the batter, fold in the beaten egg whites.

Flavor choices: Add any of these to either yogurt or rice pancakes:

Up to 1 t. ground cinnamon or nutmeg
Up to 2 t. ground coriander

GRAIN & VEGETABLE BREAKFAST

1 cup grain (any kind allowed)
2 cups liquid (chicken or turkey stock, vegetable stock or water)
1 cup finely chopped vegetables: celery, peapods, carrots, green
    beans, broccoli, etc.
1 egg
1 to 2 T. olive oil (optional)
1/4 t. celery salt
1/4 t. Mrs. Dash seasoning
1/8 t. pepper
1/4 t. garlic powder

Add the grain to boiling liquid. Bring to a boil, then reduce heat to a simmer. Cook for 30 to 35 minutes. During the last 2 minutes of cooking, add the vegetables. When all the liquid is absorbed, mix in the egg and heat through. Add olive oil (optional) and seasonings. Serves 4.

SALMON PATTIES WITH POACHED EGG

1 can drained and cleaned salmon
1 egg
1 dash of Mrs. Dash seasoning
1 T. liquid from salmon
1/3 cup rolled oats
2 T. chopped celery (optional)
8-10 poached eggs
1 small pat of butter or 1 T. olive oil

Drain salmon, save liquid. Add all ingredients except poached eggs together. Heat non-stick skillet. Add less than a pat of butter (or use olive oil) to skillet. Put a spoonful of mixture into skillet to form a pancake. Brown on both sides. Arrange on plate. Place a poached egg on top of each patty. Makes 8-10 patties.

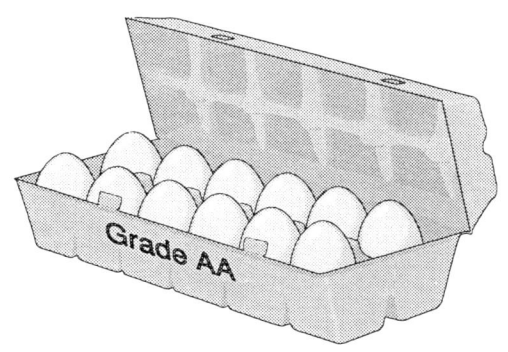

APPETIZERS

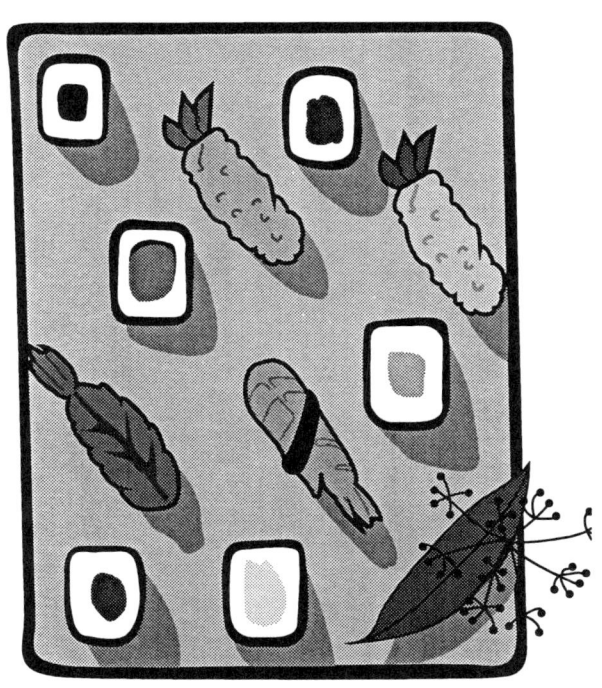

Note: Where mayonnaise is indicated, use the homemade mayonnaise recipe (p. 47) in this cookbook.

CLAMS WITH RED PEPPER MAYONNAISE

2 shallots
1 t. tarragon
1 bay leaf
1/2 cup water
2 T. lemon juice
2 cloves garlic
32 clams, scrubbed
1 sweet red pepper
3 T. mayonnaise (p. 47)
2 T. chopped fresh parsley (garnish)

Combine the shallots, tarragon, bay leaf, water and lemon juice in a large, heavy-bottom saucepan. Add the garlic by pushing it through a garlic press into the pan. Bring to a boil and add clams. Reduce heat and simmer, covered, until the clams are open, about 8 to 10 minutes. Remove clams from their shells and keep warm. Reserve half of the shells.

Roast the pepper under a broiler for 8 to 10 minutes. Put the pepper in a paper bag and allow it to sit for 30 minutes, then peel off the skin.

In a food processor or a blender on medium speed, puree the pepper. Combine the pureed pepper with the mayonnaise in a large bowl. Toss clams with the mayonnaise mixture until all are coated. Place one clam in each shell half. Garnish with parsley, if desired, and serve.
Makes 4 servings.

RUSSIAN MINTED MEATBALLS

1 1/2 lbs. ground turkey
2 eggs, beaten
3/4 cup rolled oats
2 medium onions, minced
1/4 cup minced fresh parsley
1 T. minced fresh mint
1/4 t. cinnamon
1/4 t. ground allspice
2 T. chicken stock
1 bunch parsley (garnish)

Combine the meat, eggs, oats, onions, parsley, mint, cinnamon and allspice in a large bowl. Cover and refrigerate several hours or overnight. Form the meat mixture into bite-size meatballs. Sauté half the meatballs in half the stock until browned. Keep warm. Repeat with the remaining meatballs. Serve with toothpicks, garnishing the serving plate generously with parsley, if desired.

GUACAMOLE (Avocado Dip)

1 or 2 T. mayonnaise (p. 47)
1 ripe avocado
1 T. lemon juice
1 to 3 T. minced onion
1 t. dry mustard
1/4 t. ground coriander
dash cumin

Mash the avocado with the lemon juice and onion. Stir in mustard and rest of ingredients. Serve with raw vegetables.

SPINACH SURPRISE DIP

2 cups fresh chopped spinach (chopped very fine)
2 cups parsley (finely chopped)
1/2 cup mayonnaise (p. 47)
1 cup green onions, including tops, finely chopped

Mix all together and serve with fresh vegetables.

NOTE: I have made this dip several times for company and
EVERYONE asks for the recipe. It is much better to make it up
a day or two ahead and let the flavors blend together. Can also
be made with yogurt.

SALMON PATTIES

2 small carrots, shredded
2 green onions chopped
1 egg, beaten
1 7-ounce can red salmon, drained and flaked
dash of thyme
dash of tarragon
1/2 t. parsley
lemon wedges (garnish)
parsley sprigs (garnish)

Combine the carrots, onions, and egg in a medium-size mixing
bowl. Remove any skin from the salmon, remove the bones,
and add along with the salmon meat, thyme, tarragon and parsley to the mixture in the bowl. Stir until combined. Form into
patties. Cook on a lightly oiled skillet, turning once, or broil
(preferred) until lightly browned and cooked throughout, 5 to 7
minutes on each side. Serve garnished with lemon wedges and
parsley, if desired.

SPINACH & HERB DIP

1 package frozen spinach
3/4 cup mayonnaise (p. 47)
1/2 cup plain yogurt
1 celery stalk, chopped
1 carrot, grated
2 green onion stalks, chopped
1/2 t. Mrs. Dash seasoning
To taste: onion powder, garlic powder, celery seed, paprika, co-
    riander, thyme, marjoram, sage

Squeeze juice from frozen spinach.   Mix all ingredients together. Chill for 1 hour in refrigerator.

DUTCH TARRAGON DIP

6 T. plain yogurt
1 T. mayonnaise (p. 47)
1 T. minced sweet red peppers
1 T. minced green peppers
1 T. minced celery
2 t. minced shallots
2 t. minced fresh tarragon or 1/2 t. dried tarragon
tarragon sprigs (garnish)

In a small bowl combine the yogurt, mayonnaise, red peppers,
green peppers, celery, shallots and tarragon. Place in a serving
container, garnish with tarragon and chill before serving, if desired. Makes approximately 3/4 cup. This dip is exceptionally
good when made with fresh tarragon.

DILLED EGG SPREAD

4 hard-cooked egg whites, chopped
2 T. plain yogurt
1 T. mayonnaise (p. 47)
1/4 cup minced sweet red peppers
1 T. minced fresh dill or 1/2 T. dried dill
1/4 t. ground coriander
fresh dill (garnish)

Combine the egg whites with the yogurt, mayonnaise, red peppers, dill and coriander in a medium-size bowl. Place the mixture in a serving bowl, garnish with dill, if desired, and surround the bowl with rice crackers (available at health food stores).

SALMON MUFFINS

1 can salmon
1/2 cup rolled oats
1/4 cup broccoli, chopped
1 garlic clove, chopped
1/2 cup celery, chopped
1 egg
1/4 t. Mrs. Dash seasoning
1/2 t. lemon juice
2 T. salmon juice from can

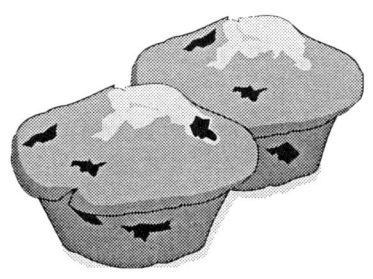

Drain salmon, save juice. Clean out bones and skin from salmon. Mix all ingredients together, except juice. Add enough juice until the mixture sticks together. Put in muffin tins that have been lightly greased with olive oil or muffin cups and bake at 325 degrees for 30 minutes.

VEGGIE MUFFINS

1 cup broccoli
1 cup cauliflower
1 green onion
2 celery stalks
1/2 cup rolled oats
1/2 cup brown rice, cooked
2 eggs, beaten
1/2 t. celery seed
1/2 to 1 t. dry mustard

Chop all vegetables very fine. Add remaining ingredients. Fill muffin tins lightly greased with olive oil or muffin cups and bake at 325 degrees for 25 minutes.
NOTE: Makes a great lunch or snack.

TUNA MUFFINS

2   9-oz. cans tuna, solid in water
1/2 cup rolled oats
2 eggs, beaten
3 stalks celery, chopped
1 green onion top, chopped
1/2 t. celery seed
1/4 t. Mrs. Dash seasoning
1/4 t. onion powder
1/4 t. garlic powder

Drain tuna, save juice. Break tuna up until shredded. Add celery and green onion. Mix well. Add remaining ingredients. Mix well. Fill muffin tins lightly greased with olive oil or muffin cups and bake at 325 degrees for 25-30 minutes.

DEVILED EGGS

4 hard boiled eggs
1/2 cup total of cooked rice and millet
1/2 t. dry mustard
1/2 t. lemon juice
1 T. green onion, chopped
1 T. celery, chopped
1 raw egg yolk

Cut eggs in half and discard cooked yolk. Mix remaining ingredients. Place in hollow egg. Sprinkle with paprika.

THIN BARLEY CRACKERS

1/2 t. baking powder
1 cup barley flour
3 T. butter or olive oil

Mix together baking powder, barley flour, and butter or olive oil. Add 1/8 t. water, or just enough to make dough you can roll out.

Roll in small shapes about 2" in diameter (circles, squares, etc.). Put in frying pan over medium high flame for about 4 minutes. Turn over and cook other side. There should be brown spots on top side and a slightly darker color when done. Let cool and put on your favorite topping such as alfalfa sprouts and sardines. Makes 15-18 crackers.

SALAD DRESSINGS & SAUCES

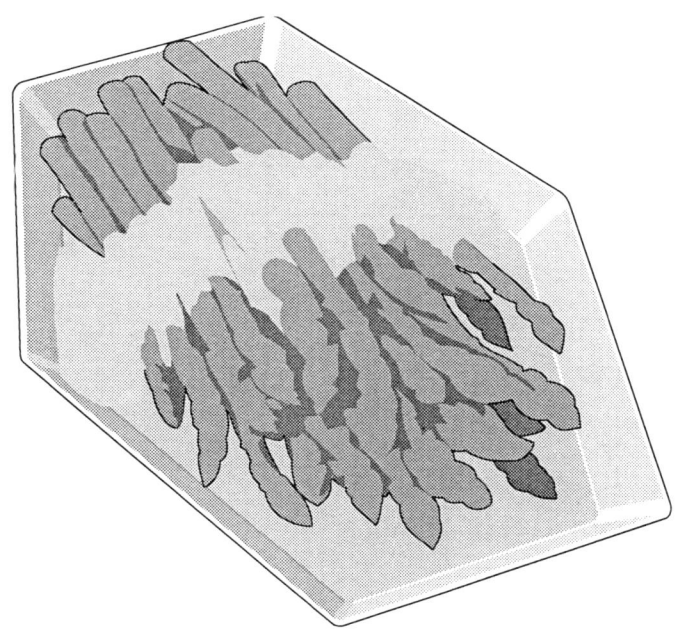

MAYONNAISE

1 egg
1/4 t. dry mustard (or more)
dash of onion powder
1 T. + 1 t. pure lemon juice
dash of salt
1 cup oil, preferably olive, flax seed, canola, or safflower

Break egg into blender. Blend on medium/high speed for 5 seconds. While still blending, add mustard, lemon juice and salt. Blend 5 seconds. While still blending, slowly add in the oil. Stick a funnel into top of blender jar to prevent splattering if your blender doesn't have the removable small center lid. It will begin to thicken after 1/2 cup has gone in. If it becomes too thick, thin with drops of water. Season to taste. Makes 1 cup of mayonnaise.

Variation: Add one beaten egg white, plus 1/4 t. dill weed to already made mayonnaise. This increases the volume and decreases the expense.

Do not double recipe. Make another batch if more is needed. Stays fresh in refrigerator for 1 week. Use this mayonnaise in any recipe in this book that calls for mayonnaise.

OLIVE OIL DRESSING

2/3 cup olive oil
1/2 t. dry mustard
1 t. celery seed
1 T. lemon juice
2 T. water
2 t. Italian herbs
garlic clove, pressed

Mix well in blender. Store in refrigerator.

Use over chicken, or for a dip for vegetables or for a salad dressing.

BASIC WHITE SAUCE

1/3 cup olive oil
3 T. barley flour
1 cup broth (see Soup section)

Warm oil on low burner. Add flour to make a paste. Stir over medium heat for a minute. Add broth. Turn heat to medium high. Stir until thickened. If too thick, add more liquid.

Use on meats, vegetables, or grains.

BROWN GRAVY

1/3 cup olive oil
5-6 T. barley flour
2 cups broth
2 garlic cloves (optional)
salt to taste

Warm oil and pressed garlic on low burner. Add flour. Stir over medium-high heat until browned. Add broth. Stir until thickened. Fantastic over turkey!

YOGURT-MAYO DRESSING

2 cups plain yogurt
1 cup mayonnaise
1 T. dill weed
1 t. freshly ground pepper
1/2 t. dry mustard
1/2 t. paprika
1/2 t. garlic powder

Mix all ingredients. Use as a salad dressing or as a dip for fresh vegetables.

CURRIED MAYONNAISE DRESSING

1 egg
1/2 t. curry powder
2 T. pure lemon juice
1/2 cup olive oil
1 clove garlic, chopped

Place egg, curry powder, garlic, lemon juice and 1/4 cup oil in blender. Cover and blend on low speed for just a few seconds. Add remaining oil in a slow stream, keeping the blender on. Good on salads.

CURRIED MAYONNAISE

1 cup mayonnaise (p. 47)
1/4 t. lemon juice
1 t. curry powder

Mix together. Great for vegetable dip.

NOTE: This is our favorite dip to serve with artichokes. Figure on about 1/4 cup per person (also, per artichoke). Great over vegetables and meats.

SAUCES

Cooked zucchini blended in blender or food processor acts as a base and thickener for sauces. These sauces are good on meats and grains. Several such recipes follow:

ZUCCHINI MUSTARD

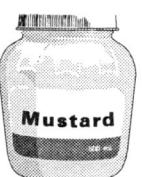

2 zucchini
Dry mustard to taste (1 T. or more)
1-2 T. lemon juice

Slice and cook zucchini. Blend until smooth in blender or food processor. Add dry mustard and lemon juice; blend.

CURRY SAUCE

2 zucchini
Salt
1/2 T. curry powder
Dash of Mexican blend seasoning or cayenne

Slice and cook zucchini. Blend until smooth in blender or food processor. Add seasonings and blend again until smooth.

CURRY SAUCE WITH NUTS

Follow directions for Curry Sauce, then add 1/3 cup pecans to blender. Blend again until smooth, adding water to thin if necessary.

MILD INDIAN SAUCE

1 zucchini, cooked and blended
1/3 cup pine nuts (pignolias)
Dash of cinnamon and nutmeg

Combine ingredients in blender; blend until smooth.

CASHEW SAUCE

1 zucchini, cooked and blended
1/2 cup cashews
1/4 t. salt

Combine ingredients in blender; blend until smooth.

MUSTARD-MAYONNAISE SAUCE

1 cup mayonnaise (p. 47)
2 T. green peppercorn mustard, or any very spicy mustard
1 t. dry mustard
1 T. parsley, finely minced
pinch cayenne pepper
2 hard-boiled eggs, finely chopped
juice of 1 small lemon

Mix all ingredients together well in a bowl and let set 30 minutes before serving. Makes 2 cups sauce. This is a wonderful sauce for cold meats.

DILLED CUCUMBER SAUCE

1/2 cup peeled, seeded and minced cucumbers
1/2 t. lemon juice
1/2 cup plain yogurt
1 t. dry mustard
1 t. chopped chives
1 1/2 t. dill

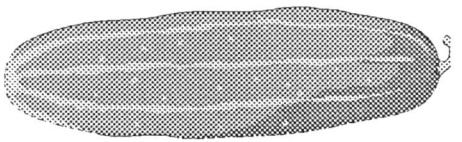

Combine all the ingre-
dients in a small bowl. Chill 2 hours before serving. Excellent
with poached salmon, as a dip for raw vegetables or as a salad
dressing.

CAESAR SALAD DRESSING

1 cup olive oil
4-6 garlic cloves, crushed (pressed)
juice from 1 whole lemon
1 can of anchovies (flat)
1 egg yolk
fresh garlic to taste

If you are healthy enough to tolerate these, add:
1 cup freshly grated parmesan cheese
1/2 t. Worcestershire sauce

Mix all ingredients together in blender.

CREAMY ITALIAN SALAD DRESSING

1/2 cup mayonnaise (p. 47)
1/4 cup olive oil dressing (p. 48)
2 T. water
1 t. Italian herbs
dash garlic powder

Mix together. Pour on favorite salad. Enjoy!

LEMON CUCUMBER DRESSING

1 cup mayonnaise (p. 47)
1 cup yogurt
1 cup cucumber, finely chopped and seeded
2 T. pure lemon juice
1 T. onion, minced
2 t. grated lemon peel

Combine all ingredients. Cover and chill 1 hour. Serve over greens. Makes 2 1/2 cups.

GREEN GODDESS YOGURT DRESSING

1/2 cup plain yogurt, mayonnaise, or a combination
1 ripe avocado
1 T. lime juice
1 t. chili powder
1 t. chopped chives, parsley or mint
1 small clove garlic, chopped

Blend all ingredients together and mix well. Makes 1 cup.

LO-CAL DRESSING

1 cup plain yogurt, mayonnaise, or a combination
1 large garlic clove, chopped
1 t. freshly chopped mint or 1/2 t. dried mint
1/4 t. white pepper
1/2 medium cucumber, peeled, seeded and finely chopped.

Combine all ingredients and mix until blended. Pour over tossed salad greens.

CLASSIC HOLLANDAISE SAUCE

4 egg yolks
3 T. pure lemon juice
1/8 t. paprika
dash cayenne pepper
1/2 cup firm butter, cut in eighths

Stir egg yolks, lemon juice and seasonings briskly over low heat. Add half the butter and stir over very low heat until butter is melted. Try not to brown butter. Add remaining butter stirring briskly until butter is melted and sauce thickens. (Butter should melt slowly to give eggs time to cook and thicken sauce without curdling.) Serve hot or at room temperature. Makes approximately 1 cup. Serve over poached eggs.

NOTE: Leftover sauce can be stored covered in refrigerator for several days. Before serving, stir in small amount of hot water.

CREAMY CUCUMBER DRESSING

1/2 cup mayonnaise (p. 47)
1/2 cucumber, slightly chopped
1/2 t. dill
1/2 t. salt
dash of Mrs. Dash seasoning

Blend in blender for 15-20 seconds or until all cucumber is pureed.

LEMON BUTTER SAUCE

1/2 cup white sauce (p. 48)
1 raw egg yolk
3 T. butter, or 1 1/2 T. each butter and olive oil
3 T. lemon juice
sea salt
Mrs. Dash or Parsley Patch seasoning
crushed garlic (optional)

Melt butter in saucepan over low heat. Add garlic if desired. Do not let butter brown. Add lemon juice, salt, seasoning, and white sauce. Continue to heat, add egg yolk and stir until thick (1 minute). Pour over grilled fish or vegetables.

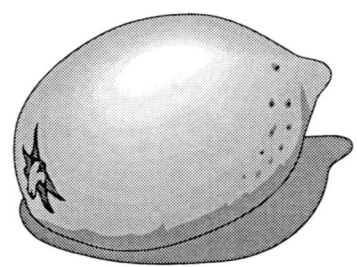

CREAMY DILL SAUCE

1/3 cup white sauce (p. 48)
1/3 cup plain yogurt
2 T. lemon juice
dill weed
sea salt

Combine white sauce, lemon juice, dill and salt. Warm on medium heat. When sauce is hot, stir in yogurt until smooth. Great on meat, rice and vegetables.

MARINADE I - FOR FISH

3/4 cup oil
1 T. lemon juice
dash dry mustard
dash onion powder
dash dill weed

Mix all ingredients together in blender.

MARINADE II - FOR CHICKEN

3/4 cup oil
1 T. lemon juice
2 T. Italian seasonings
1 garlic clove, pressed
dash of Mrs. Dash or Parsley Patch seasoning

Mix all ingredients together in blender.

YOGURT DILL CREAM

1 cup plain yogurt
3 1/2 T. finely chopped green onions, including green stems
1 T. dill weed

Mix all together and chill for several hours before serving.
Good on salads, grains, and meats.

PEGGY'S PESTO

1 cup olive oil*
2 cloves garlic
2/3 cup parmesan cheese*
2 T. pine nuts (pignolias)
3 bunches basil leaves, washed

Combine all ingredients in food processor or blender. Good on
grains and pasta.

* If parmesan cheese is not used, decrease oil to 1/2 cup.

MUSTARD

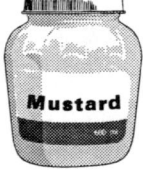

1 T. dry mustard
2 T. lemon juice
1/2 cup mayonnaise (p. 47)
Dash each onion powder and salt
Blend together. Flavor will be strong; adjust dry mustard as
needed for milder flavor.

SALADS

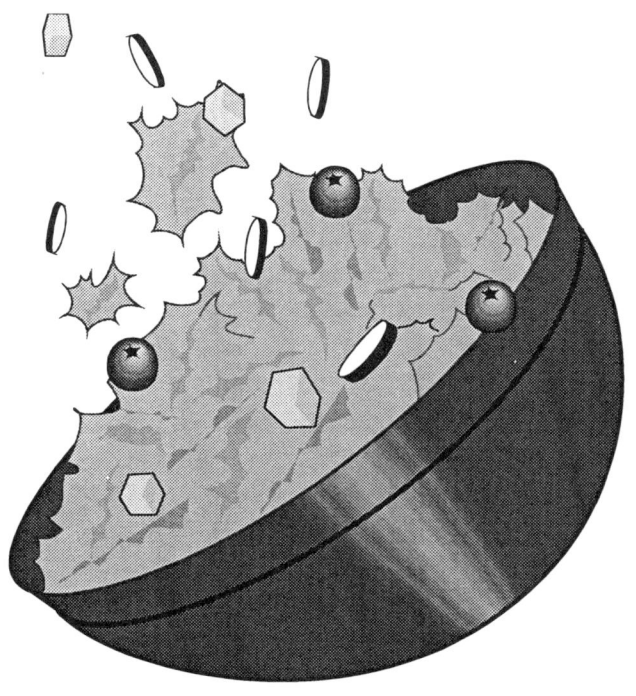

TOSSED GREEN SALAD

Romaine or Red Leaf lettuce
Cucumber, sliced
Grated carrots
Sprouts
Any fresh vegetable favorite salad ingredient allowed
Favorite salad dressing

Variations: add 1/2 cup cooled, cooked brown rice alone or with chicken, tuna, or salmon.

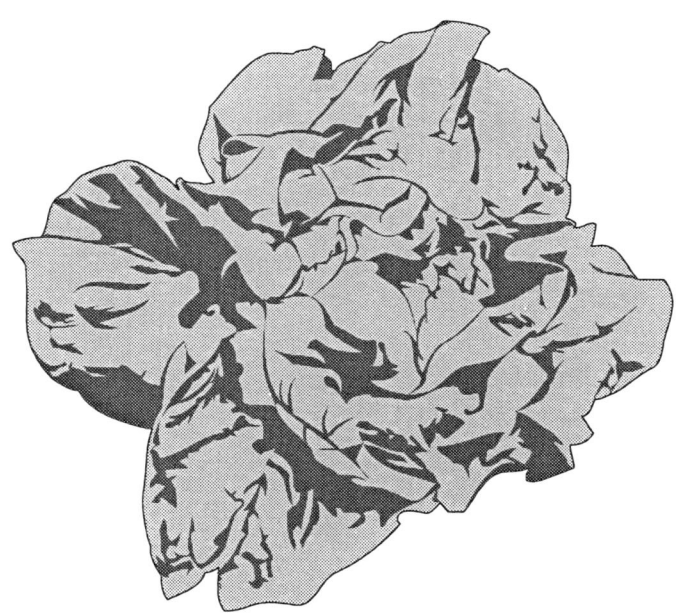

VEGGIE-POTATO SALAD

5 medium potatoes, cooked
4 hard-cooked eggs (no yolks)
1/4 cup mayonnaise (p. 47)
1 T. celery seed
1 T. paprika
1 T chopped chives
2 T. chopped fresh parsley
1/4 cup plain yogurt
2 cups chopped vegetables - any combination of the following:
    fresh spinach, raw zucchini, celery, alfalfa sprouts, green on-
    ion, cucumber

Dice potatoes and eggs and mix together. Add mayonnaise, yogurt, seasonings and your choice of vegetables. The raw things
give this salad a special crispness.

POTATO AND EGG SALAD

1 lb. potatoes, cubed
3 boiled eggs, diced (no yolks)
1 head of lettuce, shredded
1 package fresh peas (frozen OK if urine
    pH is between 5.5 and 7)
1/2 cup olive oil
1 t. dry mustard
1/2 t. sea salt
1 t. lemon juice

Combine potatoes, eggs, lettuce and peas. Mix mustard with olive oil, lemon juice, and salt. Pour over the rest of the ingredients and mix well.

EGG SALAD

Use as many hard-cooked eggs as needed for the size of the crowd. Plan on at least 2 eggs per person. Cut eggs in half lengthwise. Combine egg yolks with mayonnaise (p. 47), avocado or yogurt and mix in any of the following you like: sesame seeds, chopped green pepper, chopped green onions, any kind of fresh sprouts, chopped celery, dry mustard. Spoon mixture into egg white halves.

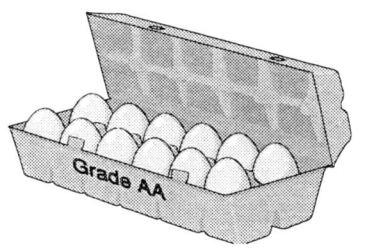

FATTOUSH SALAD

1/2 romaine lettuce, shredded
1/2 iceberg lettuce, shredded
1/2 bunch mint, minced
1 green pepper, diced
1 bunch green onions, diced
1 lb. tomatoes, diced
1 cucumber, diced
1/4 cup olive oil
Juice of 3 lemons
Pita bread or flour tortillas, or wheat-free crackers

Cut the pita bread or flour tortillas into small pieces and toast in the oven at 250 degrees until light brown. Combine all ingredients in a large bowl and mix well.

RICE SALAD

3 cups cooked brown rice
1/2 cup sliced celery
1/4 cup chopped onion
1/4 cup chopped fresh parsley

Optional:
2 to 3 cups chopped vegetables (carrots, peppers, peas, zucchini, etc.)
1/2 to 1 cup cooked poultry or fish

Dressing:
1/2 to 3/4 cup yogurt-mayonnaise dressing (p. 49)

Combine salad ingredients along with any optional ingredients you wish. Mix dressing; pour over salad. Stir and chill. Garnish with parsley if desired.

BROCCOLI SALAD

1 bunch broccoli (raw and cut into bite size pieces)
1 cup diced celery
3 hard-cooked eggs (no yolks)
1 small red onion, chopped
juice of 1/2 lemon
1 cup or more of mayonnaise (p. 47)

Mix all ingredients and chill before serving.

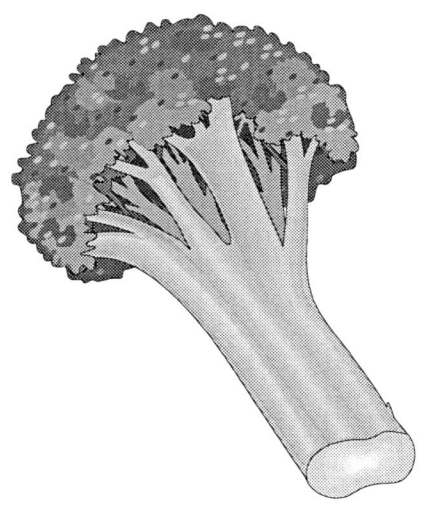

CRUNCHY CHICKEN SALAD

2 cups cooked, diced chicken
2 cups cooked brown rice, cooled
1/2 cup chopped green onion
1/3 cup oil plus lemon juice to make 1/2 cup of liquid
1/2 cup chopped celery
3/4 cup mayonnaise (p. 47)
1/2 cup chopped green peppers
dash of pepper

The night before mix cold rice, onion, oil and lemon juice. Chill overnight. Prepare remaining ingredients except green peppers and refrigerate. The next day combine ingredients. Add peppers. Add mayonnaise as needed. Chill at least 2 hours. Serve over chopped spinach leaves.

YOGURT SALAD

2 cups yogurt
1 cucumber, chopped
2 cloves garlic
1 t. dried mint

Mix the yogurt well. If too thick, add water until desired consistency. Add cucumber and then squeeze the garlic through a garlic press over the yogurt. Mix well and add the mint.

DANDELION IN OLIVE OIL

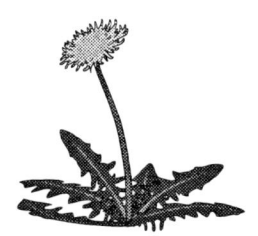

1 lb. dandelion
1 onion, chopped
3 cloves garlic
1 bunch cilantro, finely chopped
2 T. olive oil

Cut dandelion into one inch pieces and boil in water, or steam until a bit tender. Put in strainer and let cool. Squeeze out all the water and chop finely.

Put onion in skillet, add 3 T. water and simmer until tender. Add dandelion and cook for 5 minutes. Add cilantro, olive oil, and garlic and cook for five minutes longer. Serve cold or hot. Lemon juice may be added if desired.

POTATO SALAD

1 lb. boiled potatoes, cubed
1/2 bunch parsley, coarsely chopped
1 onion, diced
2 cloves garlic, minced
1/2 bunch fresh mint, minced
Juice of one lemon
1/2 cup olive oil

Combine all ingredients except olive oil. Mix well and then add the olive oil.

CREAMY SALAD GEL

1 envelope unflavored gelatin
1 cup cold water
2 T. pure lemon juice
1 1/4 cup mayonnaise (p. 47)
1 t. dry mustard
2 T. minced onion

Salad ingredients:
1 1/2 cups tuna OR 1 1/2 cups cooked chicken, OR 1 1/2 cups hard-cooked eggs (no yolks), OR 1 1/2 cups chopped seafood
3/4 cup celery, chopped
1/4 cup diced pimiento

Sprinkle gelatin over cold water in a small saucepan. Place over low heat and stir constantly until gelatin dissolves (until there are no visible granules), about 3 minutes. Remove from heat. Cool slightly. In mixing bowl gradually blend dissolved gelatin and lemon juice into mayonnaise. If necessary, beat with rotary beater until smooth. Add dry mustard and onion. Mix well. Chill, stirring occasionally, until mixture thickens slightly. Stir in prepared salad ingredients. Turn into a mold and chill until set. Serves 4.

DILLED CUCUMBER SALAD

2 cups cucumbers, diced
2 T. radishes, sliced
1/2 cup plain yogurt
2 t. lemon juice
1/4 t. ground cardamom
1/4 t. dill

Place cucumber and radishes in a bowl. In another bowl combine yogurt, lemon juice and seasonings. Mix well and pour over cucumbers. Refrigerate at least 1 hour before serving. Makes 6 servings.

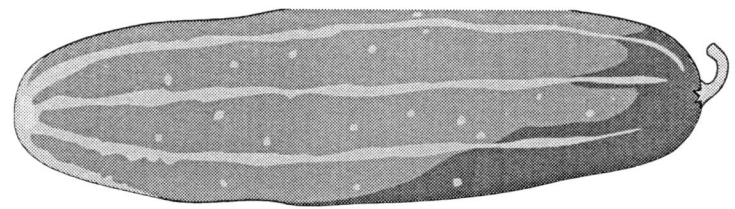

HERBIE SALAD

1 cup cooked shrimp, washed and drained
1 lb. green beans
1 medium zucchini, sliced
2 stalks celery, chopped
2 green onions, chopped
2 hard-cooked eggs (no yolks)

Dressing:
Olive oil dressing (p. 48)

1/2 head each Romaine and Boston lettuce
1/2 cup alfalfa sprouts
Chopped fresh parsley

Steam green beans until just tender, about 5 minutes. Drain, cool with cold water, and pat dry. Steam zucchini for 2 to 4 minutes. It should still be crunchy. Drain and dry. Mix vegetables with shrimp. Toss vegetable mixture with 1/2 cup of olive oil dressing. Add eggs; toss again. Chill 1 to 2 hours. Line a salad bowl with lettuce and sprouts. Add vegetable mixture. Sprinkle with parsley. Add more dressing, toss.

JELLIED CHICKEN SALAD

2 cups cut-up chicken meat from about 4 cooked chicken
    breasts
1 T. unflavored gelatin
1 1/2 cups chicken broth
1 cup mayonnaise (p. 47)
1 cup plain yogurt
1 T. lemon juice
3/4 t. dill weed
Dash of pepper (white if possible)
3 T. minced green onion
1 cup minced celery
Paprika to garnish

In saucepan soften gelatin in broth. Heat, stirring to dissolve.
Cool. Combine mayonnaise, yogurt, lemon juice, dill weed and
pepper in large bowl. Slowly stir in gelatin broth. Fold in
chicken, onions and celery. Mix well. Season to taste. Chill 1
to 2 hours, until mixture mounds slightly. Stir occasionally
while in refrigerator. Watch carefully as it begins to set around
edges - you do not want it to set in the bowl. Turn mixture into
a bowl lined with greens. Sprinkle with paprika. Chill until
firm.

MARINER'S SALAD

1 lb. cooked white fish (such as cod or haddock), cut into 1 1/2
    inch chunks
3/4 cup shredded spinach
1/4 cup julienned carrots
1/4 cup minced scallions
1/3 cup plain yogurt or 1/3 cup mayonnaise (p. 47)
1 T. lemon juice
1 T. chopped fresh parsley
1 clove garlic
1 lemon, sliced (garnish)

In a large bowl gently combine the fish, spinach, carrots and
scallions. In a small bowl, combine the yogurt, lemon juice and
parsley and add the garlic by pushing it through a garlic press
into the bowl. Pour the dressing over the salad and toss gently
until all the pieces are covered. Mound on a serving dish and
arrange lemon slices around the edges, if desired. Chill and
serve.Makes 4 servings.

TABOULI SALAD

1 cup bulghur (if allergic to wheat, use quinoa
   or steel cut oat groats)
2 bunches parsley, finely chopped
1/2 bunch mint, finely chopped
1 lb. tomatoes, diced (eliminate if sensitive)
1 bunch green onions, diced
Juice of 2 or more fresh lemons
3/4 cup of olive oil
1 t. salt
Romaine lettuce leaves

Soak bulghur in water for 1 hour before preparing. Combine bulghur, parsley, mint, tomatoes, and onion in a large bowl. Add lemon juice and olive oil and mix well. Serve on a lettuce or cabbage leaf.

QUINOA -VIDALIA SALAD

3 cups water
2 cups quinoa
1/2 t. salt
6 T lemon juice
1/2 cup olive oil
1 cup fresh basil, cut or
   shredded into 1/2" pieces
1 cup chopped Vidalia onions
   (or Maui, Imperial, or
   other mild onion)

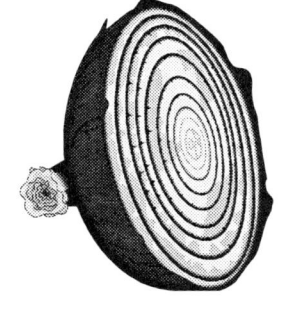

Rinse quinoa and cook in salted water for 10 minutes. Let cool slightly and add other ingredients. Mix.

MINNESOTA CHICKEN SALAD

1 whole chicken breast, boned and skinned
1 egg white
2 T. arrowroot
1 T. chicken stock
2 cups cooked brown rice
3/4 cup cooked wild rice
1 cup chopped celery
2 T. minced fresh parsley
1/4 cup yogurt-mayo dressing (p. 49)
Butterhead lettuce leaves
Grated lemon rind (garnish)

Cut the chicken into bite-size pieces. Place in a small mixing bowl with the egg white and stir to coat. Stir in the arrowroot. Allow to sit 5 to 10 minutes. Heat the stock in a medium-size skillet over medium heat, then add the chicken and cook, stirring occasionally, until the chicken is opaque throughout and lightly browned. Arrange the chicken in a single layer on a plate. Let cool for 5 minutes, then cover and refrigerate. Chill for at least 1/2 hour. In a serving bowl combine the brown rice, wild rice, celery and parsley. Add the chicken and the dressing. Serve on a bed of lettuce and garnish with lemon rind, if desired. Makes 6 servings.

COD AND CRAB SALAD

1/2 lb. cod fillet (as thick as possible)
1 1/2 cups water
1 1/2 cups chicken broth
1/2 cup mayonnaise (p. 47)
1 t. pure lemon juice
1/4 t. curry powder
1/4 t. chili powder
1/8 t. ground coriander seed
1/2 lb. fresh crabmeat (or 2 packages, 6 oz. each, frozen crab
   meat, thawed) Do not use Surimi or "Krab".
1/2 cup celery, chopped
Fresh spinach or lettuce leaves

Place cod in an 8" skillet or small saucepan and pour in enough water and chicken broth just to cover. Remove cod and bring liquid to a boil over moderately high heat. Add cod, reduce heat to low and simmer about 5 minutes until cod is opaque and will separate easily into large flakes. Remove cod from liquid. When cool enough to handle, flake fish, discarding any skin or bones. Mix mayonnaise, lemon juice, curry powder, chili powder and coriander. Toss gently with the crabmeat, flaked fish and celery. Serve on a bed of fresh spinach leaves. Serves 4.

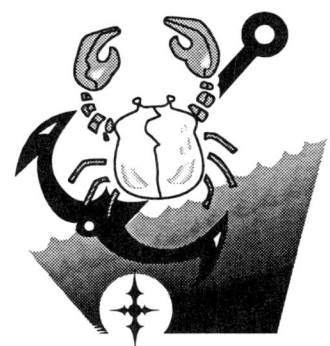

SOUPS, BROTHS AND STEWS

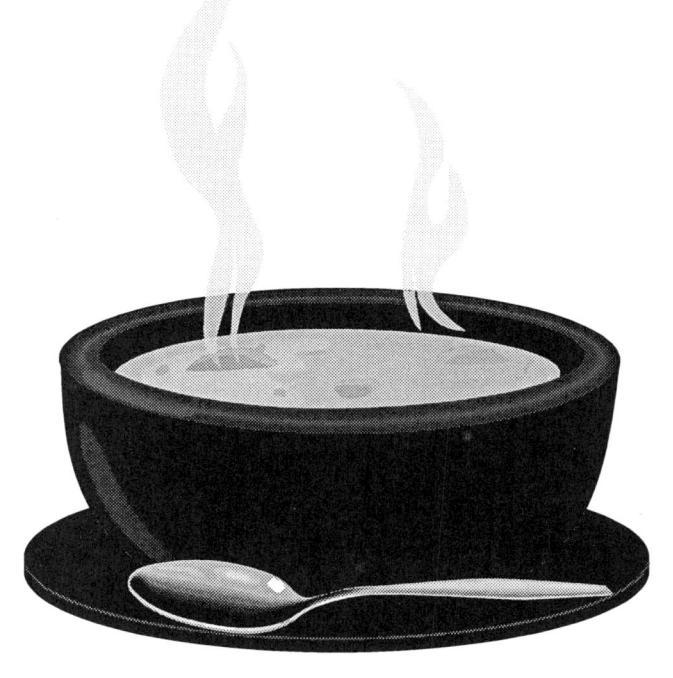

EGG DUMPLING

3/4 cup flour (not wheat - grind any grain
   of your choice with a coffee grinder)
2 t. baking powder
2 or 3 eggs, or 3 or 4 yolks
water as needed

Combine flour, baking powder and eggs. Mix until liquid is absorbed. Add water as needed to achieve doughy consistency. Drop by spoonfuls into boiling soup or stew. Lower heat and cook uncovered for 10 minutes, then cover and continue cooking for 10 minutes.

CHICKEN BROTH WITH HERBS

6 to 8 chicken pieces (or bones)
2 quarts water
tops from 6 celery stalks
1 1/2 T. Italian seasoning
2 carrots, cup up
1 stalk green onion, chopped
3 garlic cloves, chopped

Combine all ingredients in a large pot. Bring to a boil. Lower heat and simmer for 2 hours. Strain broth and freeze in containers. If chicken pieces were used, save chicken meat and discard all else.

CHICKEN BROTH

6 to 8 chicken pieces (or bones)
2 quarts water
2 to 3 garlic cloves, chopped
4 celery tops

Combine all ingredients in a large pot. Bring to a boil. Lower heat and simmer for 2 hours. Strain broth and freeze in containers. If chicken pieces were used, save chicken meat and discard all else.

SOUP STOCK

Vegetable peels and trimmings
Leftover bones, chicken necks and livers, etc. (optional)
Water to cover
A few sprigs parsley
1 or 2 bay leaves
Other seasonings to taste such as:
    marjoram, thyme, cayenne, pepper, sage, oregano, basil, garlic powder
1/4 cup lemon juice if previously-cooked bones are used (adds flavor and slows fermentation)

Collect vegetable scraps and bones as you go and store in plastic bags in the freezer until you have at least 2 quarts. Combine all ingredients in 3 to 4 quart pot. Bring to a boil; simmer for 2 hours. Strain; discard solids. Adjust seasonings and cool. Stock can be put into freezer containers for future use.

CREAM OF CELERY SOUP

Leaves, ends and trimmings
   from 1 bunch celery, chopped
1 or more small onions, chopped
1/2 cup water
2 cups thin white sauce (p. 48)

Bring celery, onion and water to
a boil. Simmer until just tender.
Puree in blender. Add more wa-
ter if needed to make 2 cups. Stir in white sauce; heat to boiling
point. Thin with additional water, if needed. If celery yields
more than 2 cups puree, add another cup of white sauce for each
cup of puree.

BASIC ORIENTAL STOCK

2 lbs. chicken bones
8 cups water
2 1/4-inch slices ginger
1 cup shredded Chinese cabbage
2 cloves garlic

Place chicken bones, water, ginger and cabbage into a large pot.
Add the garlic by pushing it through a garlic press into the pot.
Bring to a boil and skim off any foam that rises to the surface.
Reduce heat, cover and simmer gently for 2 hours. Strain and
refrigerate overnight. Remove fat from surface and refrigerate
or freeze.

QUICK EGG DROP SOUP

4 cups broth (chicken or vegetable)
1/2 cup raw brown rice
1 egg, beaten
Add anything else you want

Bring broth to boil. Add rice slowly so boiling does not stop. Cook 15 to 20 minutes. Reduce heat below boiling point; drop beaten egg in by teaspoonfuls, stirring constantly. Do not return to boil after adding egg. Makes 5 cups.

EGG DROP AND SPROUT SOUP

2 cups basic Oriental stock (p. 81)
1 egg
1 T. water
1/4 cup bean sprouts
1 T. minced fresh scallions

Bring the stock to a boil in a medium size saucepan. While the stock heats, beat the egg with the water in a small bowl. When the stock boils, begin stirring it and slowly pour in the egg while stirring. When all of the egg is added, quickly stir in the sprouts and scallions, remove from heat and serve.

WHITE POULTRY STOCK

2 pounds chicken pieces or bones (or 2 chicken carcasses)
6 cups water (or water to cover, if using carcasses)
1 cup thickly sliced carrots
1 cup thickly sliced leeks
1 cup thickly sliced celery
1/2 cup sliced turnips
1.2 cup shredded spinach
1 clove garlic
1 bay leaf
1/2 t. turmeric

Combine all ingredients in large pot. Bring to a boil and skim off any foam that rises to the top. Reduce heat, cover and simmer for 3 hours. Strain and refrigerate overnight. Remove fat from the surface; refrigerate or freeze. Makes 5 cups.

PLAIN LENTIL SOUP

2 cups lentils
6 cups water
1 onion, diced
1/2 cup rice
1/2 cup olive oil
Salt

Combine first four ingredients in a large saucepan and cook well. remove from heat, add olive oil, and salt to taste.

LENTIL SOUP WITH VEGETABLES

1 cup lentils
6 cups water
1 bunch of Swiss chard, cubed
1 large potato, cubed
1 onion, minced
2 cloves garlic, minced
2 zucchini squash, cubed
1 bunch fresh cilantro, minced
1/2 cup olive oil
Juice from 2 lemons

Cook all ingredients together in a large saucepan for 40 minutes. Add olive oil and lemon juice to soup and mix well.

If you want to keep the chard and zucchini crunchy, cook the other ingredients for 40 minutes, then add the chard and zucchini and cook together for 5-10 minutes.

VEGETABLE SOUP

10 cups liquid: 2 cups or more chicken or vegetable stock, plus
    water to make 10 cups
1 cup chopped celery
1 or 2 onions, chopped
1 small green pepper, chopped
2 T. oil, if no meat is added
2 small zucchini, diced (about 2 cups)
1 cup sliced or diced carrots
1 or 2 large potatoes, unpeeled, diced
2 cups fresh pea pods
1 or 2 cups shredded cabbage

Optional:
1/4 to 1/2 cup barley
1/2 cup raw brown rice (1 cup cooked)
1/2 cup alfalfa sprouts
1 cup (or more) any raw or cooked vegetables
Bits of leftover meat

Seasonings to Taste:
Basil, paprika, bay leaf, pepper, garlic powder, marjoram

Combine all ingredients except cabbage, barley, rice and leftovers in an 8 quart pot. Bring to a boil. Simmer, covered, for 1
to 2 hours or longer, adding remaining ingredients for the last
30 to 45 minutes. Check occasionally and add a little boiling
water if necessary. Discard bay leaf if used. Makes 6 quarts.
Recipe may be halved. Fewer vegetables may be used if you
prefer.

Slower cooker method: cook soup in slow-cooker on high for 6
hours. You may have to reduce quantities to fit cooker.

ZUCCHINI POTATO SOUP

2 or 3 medium zucchini
2 or 3 medium potatoes
1 large onion
4 cups broth (chicken or vegetable)
1 garlic clove, minced
dash of pepper
3/4 cup plain yogurt, to garnish
dill weed or curry powder to taste

Slice vegetables. Simmer in broth with garlic and pepper until tender. Puree in blender in batches. Serve hot or cold, garnish with a dab of yogurt and dill or curry. Freezes well. For a change use 1/2 bunch broccoli or 1/2 lb. spinach in place of zucchini.

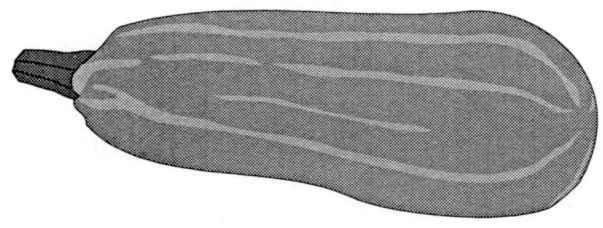

CHICKEN STEW

2 to 3 lbs. chicken, cut up and skinned
1 large onion, chopped
3 to 4 stalks celery, chopped
2 t. oregano
Dash of pepper
3 or 4 potatoes, in chunks
3 or 4 carrots, in chunks
Water to cover

Egg dumpling recipe (p. 79)

Bring chicken, onion, celery and seasonings to boil in water. Simmer about 2 hours. Remove and bone chicken, returning meat to stock. Add potatoes and carrots. Bring to boil; reduce heat to simmer until vegetables are tender. If thicker stew is desired, remove some stock, let cool, and make a gravy with flour. Return gravy back to stew and mix well.

Follow dumpling recipe and spoon into stew 20 minutes before stew is ready.

ASPARAGUS SOUP

1 lb. asparagus, cut in 1" pieces
4 cups chicken broth (p. 80)
2 t. basil leaves
2 egg yolks
4 oz. plain yogurt

Steam asparagus for 8-12 minutes. Put in blender with 1 cup chicken broth and basil, and puree. Put in pan with 3 more cups chicken broth and slowly heat. Add egg yolks and stir. Bring to simmer stirring until slightly thickened. Add other seasonings as desired. Add yogurt to each soup bowl as a garnish.

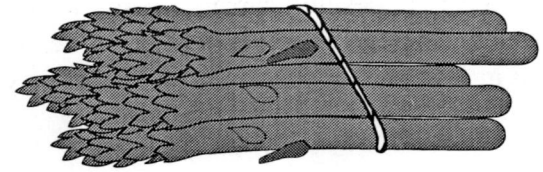

CURRIED RED LENTIL AND SPINACH SOUP

10 cups water
2 cups red lentils
1/2 cup celery, chopped
1 onion, chopped
1 t. salt
1 1/2 t. mild curry powder
1 t. cumin
1 t. garlic powder or 3 cloves chopped garlic
2 T. dried basil
1 bunch spinach, washed
juice of 1 lemon

Boil water in 4 quart pot. Add lentils, onion, celery, and seasonings. Cook 30 minutes. Add spinach and cook 5 more minutes. Remove from heat and add lemon juice.

SPINACH STEW

Lean ground meat or turkey
1 lbs. spinach, coarsely chopped
1 bunch cilantro
3 garlic cloves
1/2 t. coriander
salt

Wash spinach well. Cook meat or turkey without olive oil or butter until well cooked. Add spinach, mix well, and let cook for 10 minutes. Add coriander, cilantro, and garlic and cook another 5 minutes. Salt to taste. Serve with rice.

VEGETABLE STEW

1 eggplant (avoid eggplant if you have arthritis)
3 carrots
1/2 lb. green beans
3 squash
3 potatoes
1 onion
1 cup broth (beef or chicken)
1 lb. ground meat or turkey
1 t. oregano or basil
1 t. salt

Cut all vegetables into small pieces. Add vegetables, broth, oregano or basil, and salt to the meat or turkey and mix well. Put into a deep glass baking dish and bake at 350 degrees for 30-40 minutes.

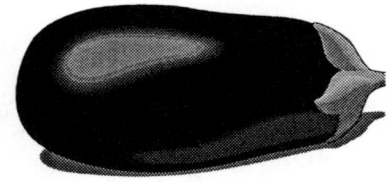

GRAIN
DISHES

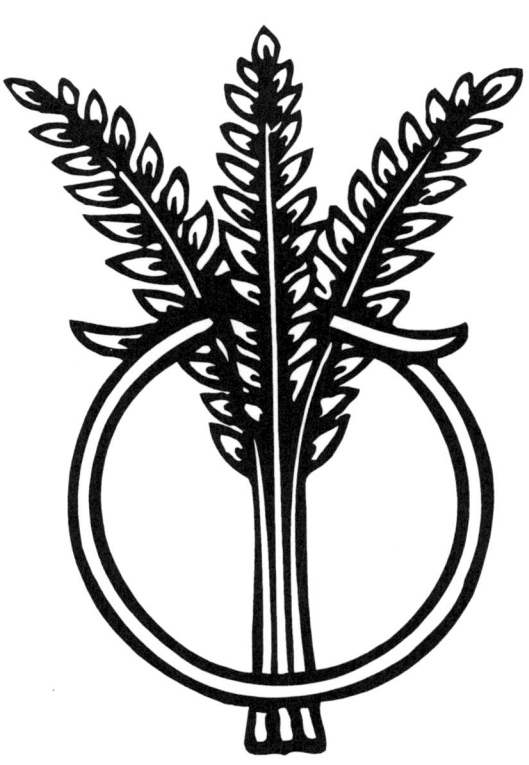

CALICO RICE

1 T. chicken stock (p. 80)
1 small onion, minced
1/2 cup shredded carrots
1/4 cup minced celery
1 cup brown rice
2 1/4 cup chicken stock (p. 80)
dash of ground cloves

Place the 1T. of stock in a medium-size saucepan and add onions. Cook over low heat until the onions are translucent. Add
the carrots and celery and cook, stirring over low heat for about
5 minutes or until tender. Add the rice, stock and cloves. Stir.
Bring to boil, then cover and turn the heat down very low.
Cook for 30-35 minutes, or until rice is tender and liquid has
been absorbed. Remove the pan from heat and let stand, covered, for about 5 to 10 minutes before serving.

FRIED RICE

3 cups brown rice, cooked
3 raw eggs, whipped with fork before adding
1 cup shrimp, cooked and chopped
1 cup peas
1/2 cup green onions, chopped
1 to 2 T. olive oil

Combine all ingredients except oil and heat on low, stirring
constantly until hot and eggs are cooked. Add oil. Serve immediately. Serves 6.

NOTE: Any vegetables can be used. Steam them for 3 minutes
to soften them.

GRAIN PILAF

1 onion, chopped
1 garlic clove, minced
2 T. oil
1 cup any grain
2 cups liquid (stock or water)
Dash of pepper

Optional:
1/2 to 2 cups chopped vegetables (celery, peppers, zucchini, sprouts, etc.)
1/2 t. oregano and/or basil
1/2 t. chili powder
1 cup leftover meat

Steam-fry onion, garlic and optional vegetables in water, keeping just enough water in pan to keep food from sticking to pan. Add grain, stirring. Add liquid and spices. Bring to a boil. Cover, simmer until grain is tender and liquid is absorbed (about 20 to 25 minutes). Stir in oil, and meat if desired.

LEMON RICE WITH VEGETABLES

1 cup brown rice, raw
1 egg, beaten
1 1/2 cups chicken stock (p. 80)
1/2 cup lemon juice
1/2 sweet red pepper, chopped
1 small carrot, thinly sliced
3 scallions, chopped

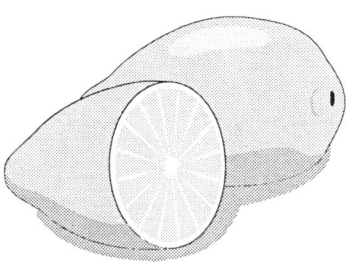

Place the rice and egg in a large, heavy-bottom saucepan and stir together. Turn the heat to medium and continue to stir the rice until the grains are separated and dry. Add the stock, lemon juice, peppers, carrots and scallions and bring to a boil. Reduce heat and simmer for 4 to 5 minutes, then cover. Turn the heat to the lowest setting and cook for 30-35 minutes, until rice is tender and liquid has been absorbed. Remove from heat and let stand 5 to 10 minutes before fluffing the rice with a fork and serving.

RICE PAPRIKASH

1 cup brown rice
2 cups chicken stock
1 small onion, chopped
1/2 sweet red pepper, chopped
1 1/2 t. paprika

Place all ingredients in a large saucepan. Bring to a boil, then reduce heat and simmer for 4 to 5 minutes. Cover and turn heat to lowest setting. Cook for 30 minutes or until the rice is tender and the liquid has been absorbed.

MILLET CROQUETTES

1 cup cooked millet
1/4 cup minced red onions
1/4 cup shredded carrots
1 clove garlic, minced
1 egg
1/2 t. marjoram
1/2 t. thyme
1 t. chopped fresh parsley
3 T. chicken stock (p. 80)

Sauce:
2 T. lemon juice
1/4 t. dry mustard
1/2 t. minced fresh parsley
1 T. mayonnaise (p. 47)

To make croquettes: Combine millet, onions, carrots, garlic, egg, marjoram, thyme and parsley in a medium-size bowl. Heat a non-stick skillet to medium and add the stock. Divide the mixture into fourths, shape each fourth in a patty and steam-fry for 5 minutes on each side.
To make sauce: Combine the four sauce ingredients in a small bowl. Serve with the croquettes.

RICE PILAF

1/2 cup chopped onion
1 garlic clove, minced
1 cup raw brown rice
2 T. oil
2 1/2 to 3 cups liquid (stock or water)
1 t. cumin and/or curry powder

Optional:
1/2 to 2 cups sliced vegetables (celery, sprouts, peppers, etc.)
1 cup cooked poultry, cubed
3 hard-cooked eggs (no yolks), chopped
2 cups cooked garbanzo beans

Steam-fry onion, garlic, rice and optional vegetables. Add liquid, oil and spices. Bring to a boil. Simmer, covered, until liquid is absorbed (about 20 to 25 minutes). Fold in meat, eggs, beans and any other options desired. Heat through.

This recipe can make a side dish or provide a high-protein meal, depending on the amount and number of optional ingredients you use. It can have a different flavor each time you make it.

SAFFRON RICE

1 small onion, minced
2 t. chicken stock (p. 80)
1/4 t. saffron
1/4 t. ground coriander
1 cup brown rice, raw
2 cups chicken stock (p. 80)

In a large saucepan, slowly cook the onions in the 2 t. stock until translucent. Stir in the saffron and cook for about 3 minutes. Add coriander and the rice. Stir the rice until any liquid in the pan has been absorbed. Add the stock and bring to a boil. Cover and turn the heat down as low as possible. Cook for 30-35 minutes, until all of the liquid has been absorbed. Keep covered until ready to serve.

VEGETABLE RICE PILAF

1 T. olive, canola, or sesame oil
2 cups grated carrots
6 scallions, chopped
1 T. minced carrot tops or fresh parsley
1 cup brown rice
2 cups water or stock

Place the oil in a large saucepan or skillet. Turn the heat on low, then add the carrots and scallions. Cook over low heat for about 5 minutes, stirring occasionally. Add the carrot tops or parsley and the rice. Cook for another 1 to 2 minutes. Add the water or stock. Bring to a boil, then cover. Reduce heat to its lowest setting and cook for about 35 minutes, until rice is tender and liquid has been absorbed. Remove from heat and let stand, uncovered, until serving.

CURRIED BASMATI RICE

1 onion, chopped
1 clove garlic, pressed
1/2 cup peas
1/2 t. red cayenne pepper, or 1/2 green pepper, diced
1/4 t. salt (optional)
1 1/4 t. curry powder
1 cup basmati rice
1 3/4 cup water

Put all ingredients in covered saucepan and bring to boil. Simmer, covered, for 15 minutes. Add 1/8 cup slivered toasted almonds (optional) for last 5 minutes of cooking time. Serves 4.

NOTE: Try adding other spices for variety (1/2 t. sage, thyme, dill; 1/4 t. turmeric or 1/8 t. saffron).

VEGETABLE
DISHES

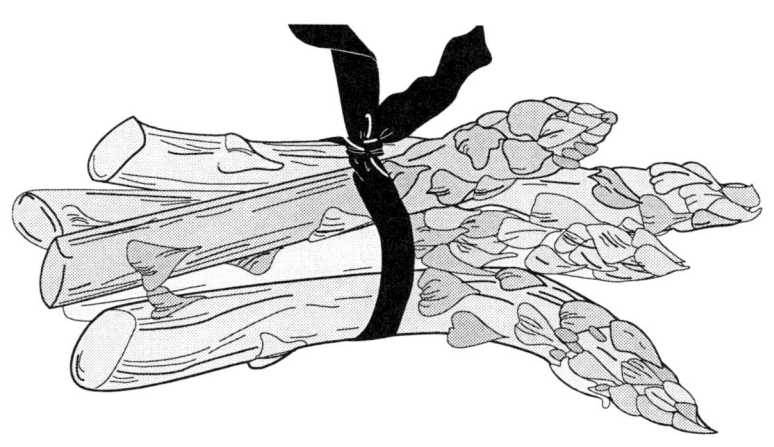

TWENTY-ONE HELPFUL IDEAS

1. Preparation is as important as the ingredients. Overcooking will dramatically decrease nutrients.

2. Leftover vegetables should be stored in glass containers--will not pick up or give off odors.

3. Serve raw vegetables with meals or as snacks.

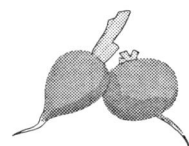 4. Next time you need a can of water chestnuts and you don't have any, try radishes! Peel off the red outside layer, steam for 5 to 6 minutes and you have your "water chestnuts"!

5. For fresh squeezed lemon juice: Roll a lemon until it's pliable. Then poke a hole in one end with a toothpick. Squeeze and out comes the juice. Replace toothpick and refrigerate.

6. Bioflavonoids are found abundantly in the white part of the lemon. Peel the yellow, leaving the white, and remove the inside of lemon. Lightly salt the white part and eat.

7. Toss lemon peels into your garbage disposal to help keep it clean and fresh smelling.

8. Spoon cold, very spicy guacamole on top of piping hot baked potatoes or grains.

9. Use broccoli stems also. Cut into large slivers, sauté or stir-fry in water until tender. At the last minute stir in a few small slices of ginger and sliced water chestnuts.

10. Chopped onions will keep for days in the refrigerator if they are rinsed and very well drained, then kept covered.

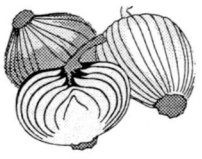

11. Steam vegetables instead of boiling them. It takes less time to steam them, so there is far more nutrient left in them than if you boil them. Also, steam them until they are still crisp, not soggy, and they taste much better, have more nutrients and won't turn to sugar as fast.

12. Save all leftover vegetables and put in freezer. When you are making soup, use these leftovers. That way you have a head start on your soup stock, and you won't have any waste. If fungus or yeast is a problem for you, it is not wise to use leftovers even if frozen.

13. When making broth always use fresh vegetables. Simmer for the appropriate time, then remove and discard the cooked vegetables.

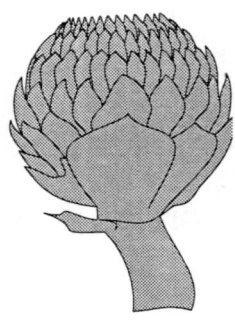

14. Try cooking your artichokes in the steamer for about 40 minutes. They come out beautifully tender and edible way up to the leaf.

15. When buying artichokes, select the smaller ones. Choose the ones with rounded, not pointed, ends. The ones with pointed ends are sometimes tougher.

16. Nutra-Fresh is a natural product that retards oxidation and browning of vegetables. Their phone number is 619-490-2855 or 619-279-3633.

17. The best way to eat vegetables is raw - more nutrients are found in them. Do not use any canned vegetables - most of them have sugar and additives in them. They are all cooked under high heat and very high pressure, thus destroying the enzymes and nutrients. If possible, avoid using frozen vegetables. Use fresh vegetables and steam them for as little time as possible to get them tender, but still crisp.

18. Do not use a pressure cooker to cook vegetables or meat. Pressure cooker means just that - high heat and high pressure - both of which destroy enzymes and nutrients.

19. To remove vegetable stains, rub hands with a slice of lemon or raw potato.

20. Always wash vegetables with Purisol, Pure Sense produce wash, or other non-toxic cleaner before using. There are many insecticides and pesticides still on them that need to be washed off, in addition to parasites and waxes on them.

21. Next time you make a salad, roast sweet or hot peppers over an open flame, turning frequently until they are very soft. Pierce with a knife to let steam escape. The skin peels off easily and the taste is smoky. Chill before cutting for salads.

SNOW PEAS AND WATER CHESTNUTS

2 cups frozen snow peas
1 cup water chestnuts*, sliced
1 T. butter
1 T. olive oil
1 1/2 t. onion powder
1 t. lemon juice
1/4 t. white pepper
1/8 t. garlic powder

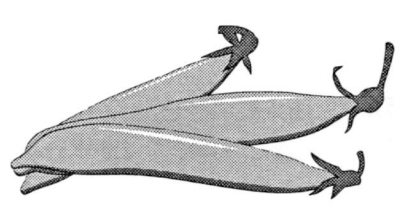

Heat water in skillet. Add snow peas and steam-fry 2-3 minutes. Add rest of ingredients. Steam for a minute until heated through. Serves 8.

*You can use "water chestnuts" made with radishes suggested in the beginning part of this section.

ZUCCHINI FLORENTINE

6 small zucchini cut into 1/4" slices
2 cups chopped uncooked spinach
2 T. butter
1 cup water
3 slightly beaten eggs
2 T. chopped onions
dash salt

Put zucchini in 1 1/2 quart casserole dish. Dot with butter. Bake at 400 degrees for 15 minutes. Combine and pour egg, water, and spinach mixture over zucchini. Set casserole in shallow pan with one inch hot water. Bake at 350 degrees for 40 minutes, until knife comes out clean.

YELLOW SUMMER SQUASH AND YOGURT

3 small yellow squash
1/2 cup chopped onion
1/2 t. paprika
2 T. fresh dill or
1 t. dried dill weed
4 t. lemon juice
2/3 cup plain yogurt (use oil recipe from p. 11 instead if allergic
    to dairy)
3 T. chopped fresh parsley

Wash squash. Cut into quarters lengthwise. Then cut into long, thin strips. In a large skillet steam-fry onion for 5 minutes. Add strips of squash, paprika, dill and lemon juice. Cover and simmer for 15 minutes, stirring occasionally. Remove from heat. Stir in yogurt. Do not reheat or yogurt will curdle. Pour into serving dish and garnish with the parsley. Makes 6 servings.

MARINATED BRUSSELS SPROUTS

2 packages (10 oz. each) Brussels sprouts or 1 1/2 lbs. fresh
1/4 cup oil or oil recipe (p. 11)
2 T. finely chopped onion
2 T. lemon juice
1 garlic clove, minced
1/2 t. dill weed

Steam the Brussels sprouts about 5 minutes. Combine remainder of ingredients and add Brussels sprouts. Mix well. Cover and chill overnight or several hours. Mix before serving. Makes 6 servings.

ORIENTAL OATS

1 to 2 cups chopped or sliced vegetables: onions, sprouts, broccoli, etc.
2 T. olive oil
1 1/2 cups rolled oats
2 eggs, beaten
3/4 cup liquid - broth or stock (p. 80)
1 cup diced meat (optional)

Steam-fry vegetables in 2 T. water. Coat oats with eggs and cook in oil until dry and separate, 3 to 5 minutes. Add liquid and vegetables (and optional meat). Simmer until liquid is absorbed, stirring occasionally.

SAVORY SQUASH

1 1/2 lbs. yellow or zucchini squash, sliced
1/2 cup onions, chopped
3 cups cooked brown rice
1 t. pepper
3 eggs, beaten
1/2 cup mayonnaise (p. 47)
Nutmeg to top

Steam squash for about 3 minutes until tender. Combine with rice, onions and seasonings. Blend eggs and mayonnaise and stir into mixture. Turn into buttered shallow casserole and sprinkle with nutmeg. Bake at 350 degrees for 20 minutes. Serves 6.

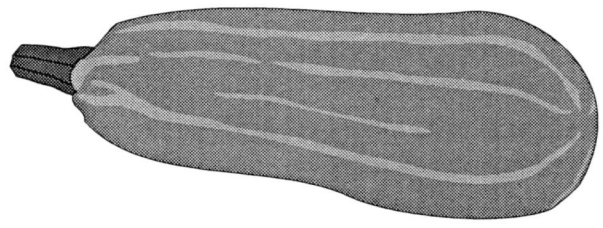

EGG AND RICE PANCAKES WITH VEGETABLE SAUCE

PANCAKE
4 eggs, lightly beaten
2/3 cup cooked rice
1/2 cup bean sprouts
2 scallions, chopped
4 t. sesame or canola oil

SAUCE
1 T. arrowroot
1 cup water
1/4 cup diced celery
1/2 cup diced green peppers
2 water chestnuts, diced
1/4 cup diced bamboo shoots
2 cloves garlic

To make pancakes: In a medium-size mixing bowl, whisk together the eggs, rice, sprouts and scallions. Heat 1 t. of the oil in a small skillet over high heat. Pour in 1/4 of the egg mixture. Turn heat to low and cook until the eggs are set, about 5 minutes. Gently turn over and brown the other side. Remove and keep warm in oven. Repeat with the remaining batter.

To make sauce: Combine the arrowroot and 1 T. water in a medium-size skillet to form a paste. Whisk in the water and place over medium-high heat. Cook, whisking constantly, until the mixture becomes syrupy. Lower the heat and stir in the celery, peppers, water chestnuts and bamboo shoots. Add the garlic by pushing it through a garlic press into the pan. Simmer for 3 minutes, stirring occasionally. Pour over the pancakes and serve.

SESAME VEGETABLES

1 T. oil
6 carrots, sliced 1/2" diagonally
6 onions, sliced
1/3 cup water
3 T. sesame seeds

Heat oil in heavy skillet. Add vegetables and sauté over medium heat for about 5 minutes, stirring frequently, or better, steam-fry. Add water and cover. Simmer until tender, about 5 to 10 minutes longer. Stir in sesame seeds and serve. The carrots and onions complement the sweetness of each other.

BAKED FRESH ASPARAGUS

3 T. melted butter
12 spears fresh asparagus
2 T. chopped onion
2 T. chopped celery
Dash of pepper

Put butter in shallow 8" x 8" baking dish. Arrange spears in dish. Combine other ingredients and pour over spears. Cover and bake at 375 degrees for 1/2 hour.

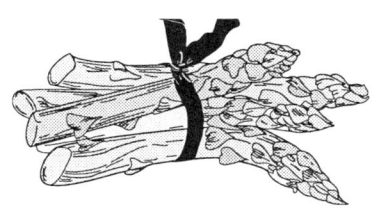

BUTTERNUT CUBES

1 butternut squash (1 3/4 lbs)
1 T. butter
1 T. olive oil
1 cup chopped fresh onion
1/4 t. dried savory
1/8 t. pepper

Steam the whole, unpeeled squash in a large kettle for 25 to 30 minutes, or until it is just tender. Cut in half and cool slightly. Pare and cut into 1 inch cubes. Melt butter in a skillet, add onion and cook about 2 minutes. Add squash cubes and seasonings and cook over low heat, stirring occasionally, for 15 minutes or until squash is tender. Serves 6.

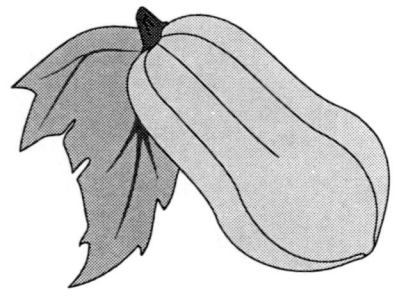

STUFFED SQUASH WITH YOGURT

1 lb. zucchini squash
1/4 cup cooked brown rice
3/4 cup meat or turkey
1 cup water
2 cups plain yogurt
1 T. rice powder
2 cloves garlic, minced
1/2 t dried mint

Remove the seeds and fibers from the inside of the squash and wash well. Combine the rice, meat, and a dash of salt and pepper and stuff the squash until 3/4 full.

Set in a pan, add 1/2 cup water and bake 30 minutes at 350 degrees or until water has evaporated. Remove from oven.

Bring 1/2 cup water and rice powder to a boil in a saucepan and stir continuously until thickened.

Remove from heat. Pour mixture over the squash and place spoonfuls of yogurt over the top. Sprinkle garlic over the yogurt and let cook for 1 minute. Sprinkle on the mint and serve hot.

EGGPLANT WITH MEAT

1 lb. meat
2 eggplants
1/4 cup olive oil
Desired herbs
Salt

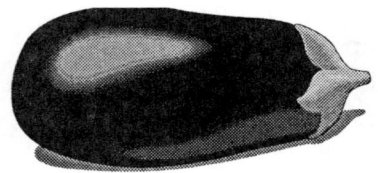

Cut each eggplant into four pieces. Dip the pieces into olive oil until coated on all sides. Broil until light brown. Set aside.

Cook meat over low heat until it is well done. Add salt and desired herbs to meat and let cool. Cut each piece of eggplant down the middle and fill with meat until well stuffed. Pour broth over the eggplant and bake in oven at 350 degrees until well done, about 20-25 minutes.

GREEN BEANS WITH OLIVE OIL

1 lb. green beans
1 onion, chopped
3 cloves garlic
2 tomatoes, diced (or use green or
    red peppers if allergic to tomatoes)
4 T. olive oil
1/2 cup water
1 t. salt

Clean the beans and cut each one into three pieces. Combine all ingredients except olive oil in a saucepan. Cook for 20 minutes. Add olive oil.

(Speed method: Decrease water and cook for 10 minutes. This method is faster but is more likely to kill food enzymes.)

CURRIED TURNIPS

2 T. oil
1 medium onion, minced
1 1/2 t. curry powder
1 cup hot chicken broth (p. 80)
2 lbs. turnips, peeled and cut into 1 inch cubes
Dash of pepper
1/2 cup plain yogurt

Sauté onion in oil until soft (or, better, steam fry) and stir in curry powder. Cook, stirring for about 2 minutes. Add 1/2 cup of the broth and the turnips. Cover and cook over very low heat about 10 minutes, or until turnips are tender. If additional broth is required, add to prevent turnips from scorching. Add a couple of tablespoons at a time so as not to have the mixture too watery. When done, the turnips should be dry. Season to taste with pepper. Remove from heat and stir in yogurt. Garnish with a dollop of yogurt and dust with paprika. Serves 6.

DILLY CARROTS

1 lb. carrots, thinly sliced
1/2 t. dill weed
2 T. butter

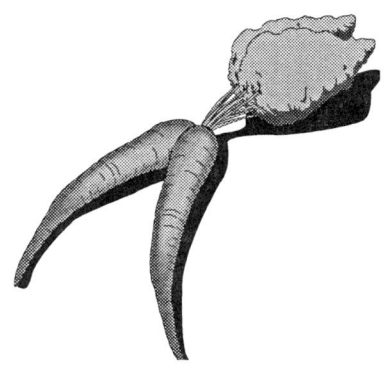

In 1-quart saucepan, steam carrots until tender, about 8 to 12 minutes. Drain. Add butter and dill. Mix well.

OKRA WITH OLIVE OIL

1 lb. okra
1 onion, cubed
2 garlic cloves, minced
2 tomatoes , diced (optional - OK if not
  allergic and urine pH is between 5.5 and 7)
1 cup water
4 T. olive oil
Salt to taste
Lemon juice

Clean okra. If cleaned the day before it will be softer. Combine okra, onion, garlic, tomatoes, water, and salt in a large saucepan. Cook for 30 minutes. Add lemon juice and olive oil.

MAIN DISHES

-

CASSEROLES

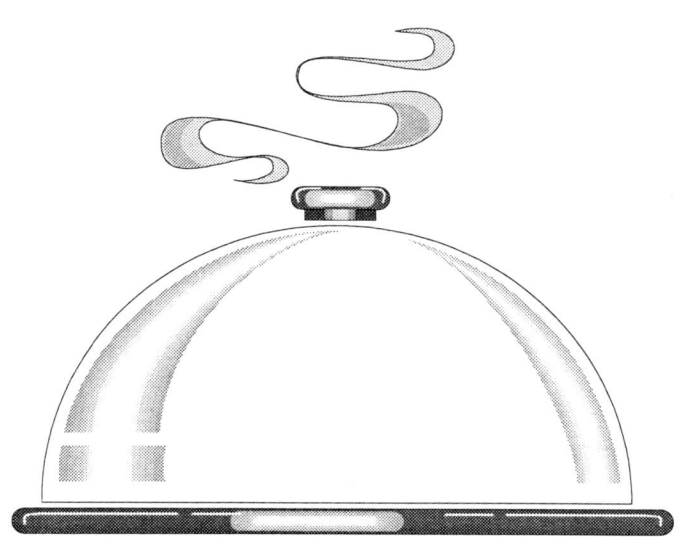

RICE AND CABBAGE

1/2 to 3/4 lb. ground turkey
1 medium cabbage, shredded
1/2 cup water
2 cups cooked brown rice

Brown meat in a large skillet. Drain fat. Add cabbage and water. Cover; simmer 7 minutes, until cabbage is crunchy but tender. Add rice. Toss lightly until well mixed.

TURKEY-ZUCCHINI CASSEROLE

2 large zucchini, cubed
1/2 to 1 lb. ground turkey
1 large onion, chopped
dash of pepper
dash of ground allspice
4 eggs

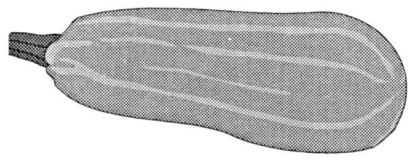

Steam zucchini. Brown turkey and onion. Drain. Add seasonings. Mix with zucchini and simmer until it is barely soft, about 7 minutes. Make 4 small wells in the mixture. Drop one egg into each well; cover pan to poach eggs.

Variation: Try adding 1/2 cup of water and 1/4 cup of millet to meat and onions. Cook for 7 minutes. All else the same.

CRAB AND SALMON CASSEROLE

3/4 cup brown rice
1/4 cup wild rice
1 medium-size onion
2 1/4 cups chicken stock (p. 80)
1/2 t. saffron
1 bay leaf
1 lemon slice
2 sprigs parsley
1/2 lb. salmon fillets
1 lb. cooked crabmeat
3/4 cup shredded carrots
1/2 cup minced green peppers
1/4 cup minced celery
1/4 cup minced onions
1 T. safflower oil
1/4 t. thyme
1/4 t. grated lemon rind
Dash of cayenne pepper
3 eggs, beaten
Lemon slices (garnish)
Parsley sprigs (garnish)

Combine the brown rice, wild rice, whole onion, stock, saffron and bay leaf in a medium saucepan. Bring to a boil, simmer for 2 to 3 minutes, then cover. Reduce heat as low as possible and cook for 20 minutes. Remove from heat and let stand for 10 minutes. Fill a small skillet 1/2 full with water and add the lemon slice and parsley. Bring to a boil, then add the salmon. Return to a boil, then reduce heat and simmer just until the salmon is cooked throughout (about 5 minutes), turning once. Drain and flake the salmon.

(continued on next page)

Remove the onion and bay leaf from the rice mixture. Combine the rice, salmon and crabmeat in a large bowl. Place the carrots, peppers, celery and onions with the oil in a small skillet and cook just until the onions are translucent. Add to the rice mixture along with the thyme, lemon rind, cayenne and eggs and stir until well combined. Place in a 9" x 13" baking dish. Bake at 350 degrees for 20 minutes, then serve hot, garnished with lemon slices and parsley.

BROWN RICE CASSEROLE

3 cups chicken broth (p. 80)
1/2 t. basil
1/2 t. thyme
1 cup brown rice, raw
2 T. oil
1 1/2 cups diced eggplant (optional)
1/2 cup chopped onion
1 garlic clove, crushed
1 cup sliced zucchini
1/2 cup chopped green pepper

In medium saucepan, heat chicken broth to boiling. Add basil, thyme and rice. Reduce heat to low. Cook covered for about 15 minutes. In medium skillet, heat oil. Add eggplant, onions and garlic. Sauté for 5 minutes. Grease casserole dish. Preheat oven to 350 degrees. Mix all vegetables, onions and garlic with rice. Pour into casserole dish and sprinkle on paprika or nutmeg. Bake, covered, for 20 minutes. Serves 6.

SPICED RICE WITH CHICKEN CASSEROLE

1 lb. chicken
5 cups water
1 stick cinnamon
1 bay leaf
1/2 t. salt

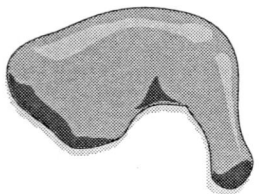

Boil chicken in water with cinnamon stick and bay leaf until tender. Remove from heat. Remove the chicken from the water and keep water as broth for the rice.

The rice:
1 lb. ground turkey or lean ground meat
2 cups brown rice
1/2 t allspice
2 t. ground cinnamon
1 t. salt
pepper to taste (use cayenne pepper
    if you have stomach problems)
1/2 cup pine nuts
1/2 cup blanched almonds

Cook ground turkey or lean meat in a skillet with 2 T. water until meat is well cooked. Add allspice, cinnamon, salt and pepper and mix well. Pour the broth remaining from the chicken over the meat and bring to a boil. Add the rice and let cook for 15 minutes. Let cook over low heat for 15 minutes longer or until water has evaporated. Put the rice on a platter and garnish with the nuts, or if you prefer mix the nuts in. Serve the rice with small pieces of chicken on top.

BARLEY VEGETABLE CASSEROLE

1 cup barley
2 1/2 cups water
1 T. oil
1 t. oregano
1 large onion, chopped
1 cup green pepper, chopped
1/2 to 1 cup any vegetable, chopped

Put barley in casserole dish. Add water. Stir well. Add rest of ingredients. Stir to blend. Bake at 350 degrees. After it has been baking for 45 minutes, stir it. Put back in oven and bake 15 minutes longer for a total of 1 hour.

CHICKEN AND RICE CASSEROLE

2 cups cooked chicken
3 to 5 cups cooked rice
1 stalk celery, chopped
1 medium onion, chopped
2 medium carrots, chopped
2 T. oil
1 t. curry powder (or less)
1 cup chicken broth (p. 80)
1 cup plain yogurt
Mrs. Dash or Parsley Patch seasoning

Sauté celery, onion and carrots in oil, or better, steam-fry. Cook for 5 minutes. Mix all ingredients together. Put in lightly oiled 9" x 13" baking pan, and sprinkle with paprika. Bake at 350 degrees for 40 minutes.

CONFETTI CASSEROLE

1 1/2 cups stock (chicken or vegetable) (p. 80)
1 cup cooked chicken, cut up
1 carrot, diced
1 celery stalk, sliced
1/4 cup onion, chopped
1/4 to 1/2 cup fresh or frozen peas
1/2 cup stock (p. 80)
2 T. arrowroot
Cooked brown rice

Add chicken and vegetables to 1 1/2 cup stock. Bring to a boil. Reduce heat and simmer until the vegetables are tender, about 20 minutes. In a small jar, combine 1/2 cup stock with arrowroot. Mix well. Add arrowroot with stock to the chicken and vegetables. Stir in well and cook until thickened. Serve over hot brown rice.

MAIN DISHES

\-

POULTRY

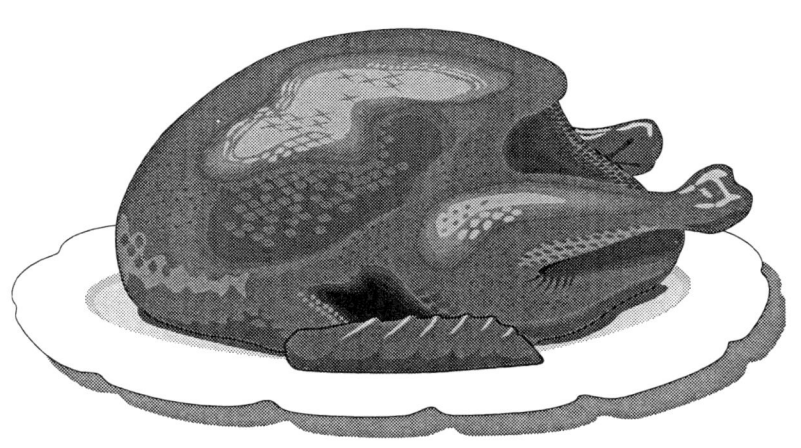

TURKEY MEATLOAF

2 lbs. ground turkey
1 green onion, chopped
1/2 cup oatmeal
1/2 t. celery seed
1/4 t. Mrs. Dash or Parsley Patch seasoning
1/4 t. coriander
2 celery stalks, chopped
1/4 t. garlic powder
1 T. mustard
2 eggs

Mix all ingredients together. Put into loaf pan and bake at 325 degrees for 1 hour.

VEGETABLE MEATLOAF

2 lbs. ground turkey
1/4 to 1/2 cup raw grated potato
1/4 cup chopped onion
1/4 cup grated carrot
dash pepper
1/2 to 1 cup liquid (broth, gravy)
1 cup chopped vegetables (optional):
    peas, green beans, celery, green peppers, sprouts, etc.

Mix all ingredients together. Bake at 350 degrees for 1 hour.

THANKSGIVING TURKEY

1 fresh turkey (Be sure to read the label carefully. Some are injected with sugar, etc. for taste enhancing.)

Prepare turkey as your tradition goes (as long as it's within the framework of your diet).

Cooking longer but at a lower temperature preserves moisture and nutrients.

TURKEY STUFFING

1 1/2 t. sage
2 t. salt
1 1/2 t. celery salt
1 t. onion powder
1 t. oregano
1/2 t. Mrs. Dash or Parsley Patch seasoning
3 cups grains
1/2 cup melted butter

Cook grains in 4 cups of water until water is absorbed. (Suggested: a combination of 1/2 cup millet, 3/4 cup oats, 1 1/4 cups brown rice and 1/2 cup wild rice.) Add 1/2 of seasonings. Add the rest to 1/2 cup melted butter. Mix all together and stuff into turkey. Bake turkey as usual.

Cook turkey once a month, stuffed or not stuffed. It's a real treat!

STEAMED CHICKEN

2 to 3 lbs. chicken parts
4 cups water
2 to 4 cups cooked brown rice

Put water into a 6 to 8 quart pot. Bring to a boil. Place chicken in steamer basket in pot. Cover tightly. Steam until tender, about 45 minutes. Serve over rice or use the boned meat in vegetable or chicken salads, as steamed chicken is more moist than roasted chicken. You can cook even a frozen chicken this way, just cook it longer, about 1 1/4 hours.

SWEET STUFFED CHICKEN BREASTS

5 to 6 boneless chicken breasts
3 celery stalks, diced
2 garlic cloves, minced
1/4 cup onion, minced
1/2 cup zucchini, diced
1 medium carrot, grated
1 t. tarragon
1/2 t. sweet basil
1/2 t. celery seed
3 T. olive oil
2 T. rolled oats

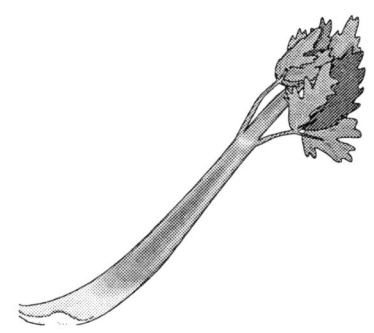

Place chicken breasts on waxed paper and pound on both sides until flat. Set aside. In saucepan, heat olive oil and add all ingredients except oats. Sauté until tender. Remove from stove. Stir in oats. Place a spoonful of mixture into center of each chicken breast. Fold breast over the mixture and secure it with toothpicks. Bake in 350 degree oven for 25 minutes.

YOGURT CHICKEN

3/4 lb. chicken breast
1 medium onion, sliced
6 small carrots, cut lengthwise into flat strips
1 cup chicken stock (p. 80)
1/8 t. celery seed
1/8 t. thyme
1/8 t. pepper
2 cups cauliflower, steamed
1 cup frozen peas
1 T. rice flour
3/4 cup plain yogurt
1 T. chopped fresh parsley

Remove skin, fat and bones from chicken breast. Cut in half-inch cubes and steam-fry until white and separate, adding water as needed to keep chicken from sticking. In large saucepan, combine onions, carrots, stock, celery seed, thyme and pepper. Bring to boil, cover and simmer 20 minutes, adding a small amount of water if necessary. Add chicken, cauliflower, and peas to saucepan. Simmer until vegetables are tender, about 5 minutes. Combine flour with 2 T. of water or stock, and stir into pot. Bring to a boil for a minute or two to thicken, stirring constantly. Remove from heat. Stir in yogurt and serve topped with parsley.

BAKED CHICKEN BREAST SUPREME

1 or 2 packages of boneless chicken breasts
1 cup plain yogurt
2 T. lemon juice
1 1/2 t. celery salt
1 t. paprika
2 cloves garlic, finely chopped
1 t. salt (or less)
1/4 t. pepper
3 WASA crackers (rye)
2 T. butter

Take skin off chicken. Wash and dry with paper towel. In large bowl combine yogurt with lemon juice, celery salt, paprika, garlic, salt and pepper. Add chicken to yogurt mixture, coating each piece well. Let stand, covered, in refrigerator overnight. Next day preheat oven to 350 degrees. Melt butter. Crush WASA crackers. Remove chicken from yogurt mixture and arrange single layer in large, shallow baking dish. If desired, you may spoon remaining yogurt mixture over chicken. Sprinkle with the WASA crumbs and spoon melted butter over chicken. Bake uncovered for 35-40 minutes or until chicken is tender and nicely browned.

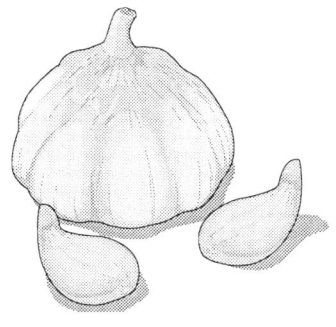

BREADED CHICKEN

5 to 8 pieces of chicken
2 T. rye flour
2 T. oat flour
2 T. Italian herbs
1 t. celery seed
1/2 t. garlic powder
1/2 t. oregano
1/4 t. salt
2 eggs
1 T. water
3 crumbled WASA rye crackers

Skin and defat chicken. Set aside. Mix dry ingredients and place in a shallow pan. Set aside. Blend eggs and water and place in a bowl or a shallow pan. Dip chicken pieces in egg mixture until well saturated. Then roll in flour mixture until coated. Place coated chicken in a pan on a rack. Bake at 350 degrees for 30 minutes, then turn over and bake for an additional 15 minutes.

CURRY CHICKEN

4 cooked chicken breasts
1 T. olive oil
2 cups vegetables, chopped:
    (zucchini, broccoli, sprouts, cauliflower, etc.)
1 cup cooked brown rice
1 t. curry powder

Sauté vegetables in oil until tender. Add remaining ingredients, mixing well. Heat thoroughly and serve immediately.

CHICKEN TARRAGON

6 to 8 pieces of chicken
2 to 3 garlic cloves
2 T. olive oil
1 1/2 t. tarragon
1/2 t. celery seed
1/2 cup water
1 T. arrowroot
1 celery stalk, chopped

Steam-fry garlic in large frying pan. Add chicken and cook for 1 minute. Add water, tarragon and celery seed. Cover and cook for 25 minutes. Add celery and continue cooking for 5 more minutes. Add arrowroot, mixed with small amount of water, to chicken and stir until thick. Add oil. Serve over hot brown rice.

MARINATED CHICKEN

5 to 10 pieces of chicken
Marinade II (p. 57)

Skin and defat chicken. Place in a pan. Pour marinade sauce over the chicken. Let set for 2 to 6 hours. Barbecue or broil for 15 to 18 minutes, turning and dipping back into sauce every 3 minutes.

LEMON CHICKEN

1 T. lemon rind, grated
1/4 cup lemon juice
1/4 cup water
1/4 cup oil
1 garlic clove, minced
1 t. pepper (or less)
1 chicken, in pieces
1/2 cup flour
2 t. paprika

Remove skin and fat from chicken and set aside. Combine first 5 ingredients plus half the pepper. Pour over chicken, cover and chill at least 3 hours or overnight. Drain chicken on absorbent paper, reserving marinade. Mix flour with remaining pepper and the paprika and use to coat the chicken. Shake off excess. Place in a shallow roasting pan and bake at 350 degrees for 30 minutes. Turn chicken over and pour marinade over it. Bake an additional 30 minutes, basting occasionally.

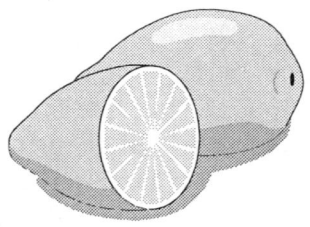

ICELANDIC MEATBALLS

1 1/2 lbs. ground turkey
2 eggs
1 cup oat flour
1/2 t. salt
1/4 t. pepper
2 t. nutmeg
1/2 t. allspice
2/3 cup water with 1 T. yogurt
1/2 to 1 cup onions, chopped

Combine in large bowl ground turkey, eggs, water with yogurt, onions and spices. Mix together lightly. Gradually add the flour and beat vigorously until smooth and well blended. Roll meat mixture into 2" balls and bake 20 minutes at 350 degrees. Serve with potatoes, cabbage or any other vegetable.

LEMON-PARSLEY MEATBALLS

1 lb. ground turkey
2/3 cup chopped parsley
2 Lite Rye WASA crackers, crushed
    (or Reva wheat-free crackers)
1/3 cup onions, chopped
1 T. yogurt blended with 1 T. water
1/4 t. salt
1/4 t. pepper
1/4 t. thyme
1/4 t. grated lemon peel
2 T. oil
1/2 cup water
1 T. lemon juice
1 T. arrowroot
Cooked brown rice

In a large bowl mix together ground turkey, parsley, crushed WASA crackers, onions, yogurt and water mixture, salt, pepper, thyme and lemon peel. Shape into 2" balls and bake 15 minutes at 350 degrees. Stir together water, lemon juice and arrowroot. Place meatballs in skillet and add sauce mixture to skillet. Bring to boil. Cook and stir 1 minute. Serve over hot brown rice. Serves 4 to 6.

CHICKEN AND DUMPLINGS

1 whole chicken in pieces, skinned and fat removed
2 bay leaves
1-2 celery stalks, cut up
3 carrots, cut up
1 small onion, cut up
1-2 garlic cloves, minced
1 egg dumpling recipe (p. 79)

Put chicken in a large 10 quart pot. Add water to cover and add bay leaves. Bring to a boil, reduce heat and simmer for 1 hour, covered. Remove chicken and all bones from stock and add vegetables. While vegetables are cooking, remove all bones from chicken and put chicken back in pot. Add more water, if necessary, to cover. Continue cooking for 30 minutes longer. While the vegetables are cooking, make the egg dumpling batter according to recipe on p. 79. Add the batter to the stew by the tablespoonful. Simmer for 10 minutes uncovered, then 10 minutes covered. When the dumplings are done, serve.

MAIN
DISHES
-
FISH

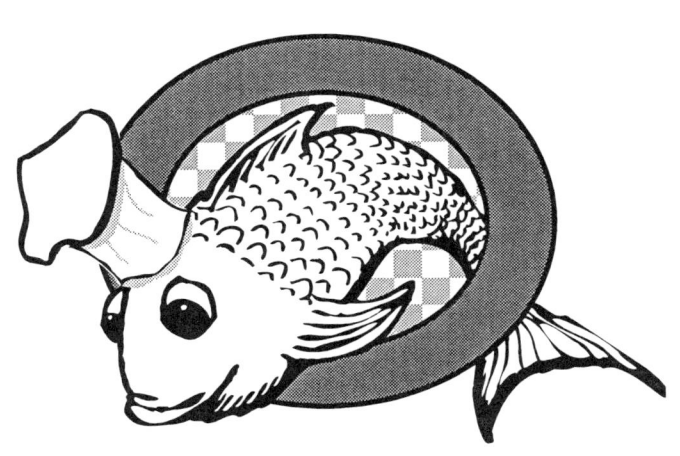

BAKED FISH FROM TURNING ISLAND

1 1/2 to 2 lbs. fish fillets
1 T. minced onion
1/2 cup mayonnaise
1/2 t. marjoram
1/2 t. dry mustard
1 t. lemon juice
Dash of pepper
Paprika

Place fish in olive-oil-coated baking dish. Mix remaining ingredients except paprika. Spread over fish. Bake at 300 degrees for 17 to 20 minutes, until browned. Sprinkle with paprika.

BAKED FISH WITH SPINACH

1 lb. fish fillets
1/2 cup flour, seasoned with pepper and paprika
2 T. butter
1 cup medium white sauce
dash of nutmeg
1 lb. fresh spinach, chopped and cooked
Dash of paprika

Cut fish into bite-sized pieces. Roll in flour, then brown in butter. Prepare white sauce. Add nutmeg. Drain or squeeze excess water from spinach. Oil a 2 quart baking dish. Arrange fish along the sides; mound spinach in the middle. Cover with sauce and then sprinkle with paprika. Bake at 300 degrees for 15 to 20 minutes.

CALICO FISH

1 lb. fish fillets
1 T. lemon juice
Dash of pepper
2 cups peas (or diced celery if prone to fungus)
1 medium carrot, grated
1 small onion, sliced and separated into rings
2 T. butter

If fillets are large, cut into 5 or 6 pieces. Arrange in ungreased baking dish. Sprinkle with lemon juice and seasonings. Spoon vegetables over fish and dot with butter. Cover and bake at 350 degrees for 20 to 30 minutes, until fish flakes easily.

FISH CAKES

2 cups tuna fish
1 cup cooked brown rice
1 egg
1 small onion, finely chopped
1 T. lemon juice
3 T. olive oil combined with 1 pat butter
WASA crackers (rye) or Reva wheat-free crackers

Beat egg and add tuna, rice, onion, lemon juice and oil/butter mixture . Blend well and form into patties. Roll in cracker crumbs and place on oiled baking sheet. Bake at 350 degrees for 15 minutes or until brown and bubbly. May substitute any cooked fish or poultry for tuna.

SKEWERED SHRIMP AND VEGETABLES

Medium to large shrimp
Green peppers, cut into large pieces
Onion, cut into large pieces
Chicken, cooked and cubed
Sea food of any kind
Marinade I (p. 57)

Marinate all ingredients in marinade sauce overnight. Skewer all pieces on skewer sticks and barbecue or broil, brushing with marinade sauce occasionally, until browned. Serve over hot rice.

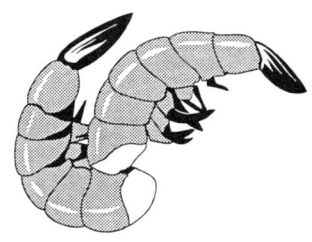

MARINATED FISH

3 to 6 fish fillets
Marinade I (p. 57)

Prepare marinade. Marinate fish for 6 hours. Broil fillets for 6 minutes, dipping into marinade sauce every 2 minutes.

Broil as follows:
    Cod, swordfish or shark--broil 6 minutes.
    Monkfish, red snapper--broil 4 minutes
Fish fillets can also be barbecued.

143

MOCK LOBSTER

1 lb. frozen cod fillets
2 onions, quartered
2 lemons, quartered
1 T. dill weed
1 T. celery seeds
1/2 t. Mrs. Dash or Parsley Patch seasoning
water to cover fish

Place fish in a large skillet and add water to cover. Remove fish and set aside. Add onions, lemons and seasonings to water. Bring to a boil and simmer for 30 minutes. Add frozen cod. Cook until cod flakes easily, about 20 minutes. Drain in colander.

SCALLOPED TUNA

12 oz. tuna, drained
2 cups medium white sauce (p. 48)
Dash of pepper (or use cayenne if stomach problems)
2 T. prepared mustard (p. 58)
3 1/4 cups cooked, sliced potatoes
1 cup chopped onion

Make white sauce. Add seasonings. Layer potatoes, tuna and onion in greased 1 1/2-quart casserole. Add sauce. Bake at 375 degrees for 45 minutes.

SALMON STEAKS WITH CURRIED AVOCADO SAUCE

4 salmon steaks (4-6 ounces each)
2 lemons, sliced
1/2 avocado
2 t. minced fresh tarragon or 1 t. dried tarragon
1/4 cup plain yogurt
1/4 t. curry powder
Tarragon sprigs (garnish)

In a saucepan filled 1/2 inch full with water, poach the salmon with 2 lemon slices over each steak until cooked through, about 15 minutes. Remove the lemon slices and place the salmon on a plate. Cool, then chill. When ready to serve, place the avocado in a blender with the tarragon, yogurt and curry. Process on low speed until smooth. Place a broad ribbon of avocado sauce across each salmon steak. Garnish with fresh lemon slices and tarragon, if desired. Serve immediately. Serves 4.

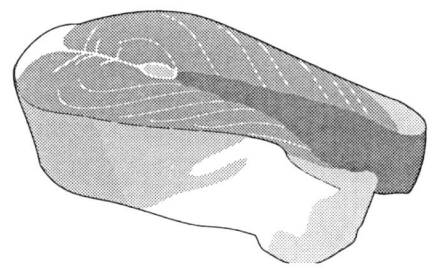

MAIN
DISHES
-
VEGETABLES

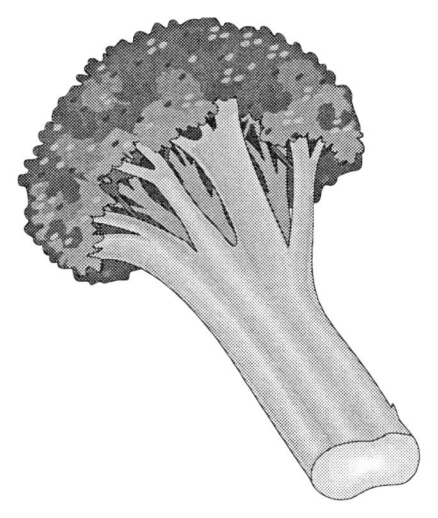

MILLET AND VEGETABLES

1/2 cup millet
1 1/2 cups boiling water
2 1/2 cups mixed raw vegetables (for example, 2 leaves of spinach torn in pieces, 3 chopped sprigs of parsley, 1/2 cup coarsely chopped onion, 1/4 cup thinly sliced cauliflower, 1/4 cup diced zucchini, 1/4 cup sliced or diced carrot, 1/4 cup sliced celery)
1 t. grated lemon peel
1 t. lemon juice
Generous pinch of saffron

In a heavy pan toast millet until lightly browned, stirring constantly. Steam vegetables. In a large casserole dish, combine millet and boiling water. Add all other ingredients and stir. Bake covered at 350 degrees for 40 minutes. Serves 6.

VEGETABLE POT

3 cups shredded cabbage
2 cups cubed potatoes
1 cup sliced carrots
1 stalk celery, sliced
1/4 t. thyme
1 cup water

Place all of the ingredients in a large saucepan. Bring to a boil, then reduce heat to simmer. Partially cover and simmer for about 30 minutes or until quite tender. Serve with the cooking liquid.

ZUCCHINI SPINACH BAKE

2 garlic cloves, peeled
2 T. plus 1 t. olive oil
1 lb. fresh spinach, washed and trimmed
3/4 lb. zucchini, diced, about 2 cups
2/3 cup onions, chopped
1 T. basil leaves
5 eggs
1/8 t. pepper

Flatten 1 garlic clove with the side of a knife. In a large, heavy saucepan or Dutch oven, warm 1 t. of the oil over moderate heat. Add spinach and the flattened garlic clove. Cover pan and cook 4 minutes, stirring 4 to 5 times, until leaves are just wilted. Drain spinach, discard garlic clove and wipe out pot. Heat oven to 350 degrees. Heat pot over moderate heat with 1 1/2 T. of the oil. Chop remaining garlic clove and mash until smooth. Add to pot with zucchini, onion and basil and cook just until onion is soft. Mix in spinach.

Grease long shallow baking dish with the remaining olive oil and spread vegetable mixture over bottom of dish. Beat eggs lightly with pepper. Pour over spinach and tilt the dish several times to distribute eggs. Bake about 12 minutes, until egg is set. Serves 6.

SHRIMP ZUCCHINI

1 1/2 cups water
1 lemon slice
1 bay leaf
1/4 lb. medium-size shrimp, peeled and deveined
1/4 cup cooked brown rice
4 small zucchini (about 6 inches long each)
1/2 cup very small broccoli florets
1 small carrot, cut diagonally into thin slices
32 snow peas
2 T. plain yogurt
2 t. mayonnaise (p. 47)
2 t. minced sweet red and/or green peppers
2 t. minced celery
1 t. minced shallots
1 t. minced fresh tarragon or 1/4 t. dried tarragon
1/2 clove garlic
Tarragon sprigs (garnish)

In a small saucepan, bring the water, lemon and bay leaf to a boil. Reduce heat, add shrimp and simmer just until the shrimp are opaque, about 3 to 5 minutes. Drain and set aside to cool.

Cut the zucchini in half lengthwise and steam for about 3 to 4 minutes or until crisp-tender. Rinse under cold water until cool. Hollow out the zucchini halves, leaving enough of the shell intact to hold their shape well. Chop and reserve removed zucchini.

Separately steam the broccoli, carrots and snow peas for about 2 to 3 minutes or until crisp-tender. Rinse under cold water until cooled. Add the broccoli to the rice in the medium-size bowl. Set aside the carrots and snow peas.

(continued on next page)

In a small bowl, combine the yogurt, mayonnaise, reserved chopped zucchini, red peppers, green peppers, celery, shallots and tarragon. Add the garlic by pushing it through a garlic press into the bowl. Stir to combine.

Chop the shrimp and add to the rice and broccoli in the medium-size bowl. Add the dressing mixture and toss until combined.

Stuff the shrimp and rice mixture into the zucchini halves. Arrange the carrot slices on top of the zucchini boats. Place each zucchini half on a small plate and arrange a fan of snow peas along one side. Garnish with tarragon sprigs, if desired. Serves 4.

SPINACH NOODLES WITH VEGETABLES JULIENNE

1/2 lb. spinach noodles (these may have wheat - avoid if wheat allergy and substitute wheat-free noodles)
4 cloves garlic, minced
1 t. minced fresh ginger
1 cup vegetable stock
1 cup shredded Chinese cabbage
2 scallions, minced, including green part
1/2 cup thinly sliced sweet red peppers
1 T. chopped fresh parsley or coriander (garnish)

Soak noodles for 20 minutes and drain. In a medium-size saucepan, combine the garlic, ginger, and stock and heat through. Add the cabbage and scallions and bring to a boil. Reduce heat, add peppers and noodles and cook until heated through. Transfer to a serving bowl and garnish with fresh parsley, if desired.

CABBAGE ROLLS I

1 medium cabbage head
1 lb. ground turkey
1/2 cup onions, chopped
1/2 cup carrots, grated
1 1/2 to 2 cups cooked brown rice
1/2 t. Italian seasoning
1/4 t. celery seed
2 cups white sauce (p. 48)

Brown meat and onions. Add remaining ingredients and mix well. Heat thoroughly. Set aside. Steam cabbage for 10 minutes. Separate leaves. Place 2 to 3 T. meat and vegetable mixture in each leaf and roll up. Put any leftover leaves and meat mixture in bottom of greased casserole dish. Lay rolled leaves, seam side down, in dish. Pour white sauce over all. Cover, bake 30 minutes at 325 degrees. Rolls can be frozen and reheated.

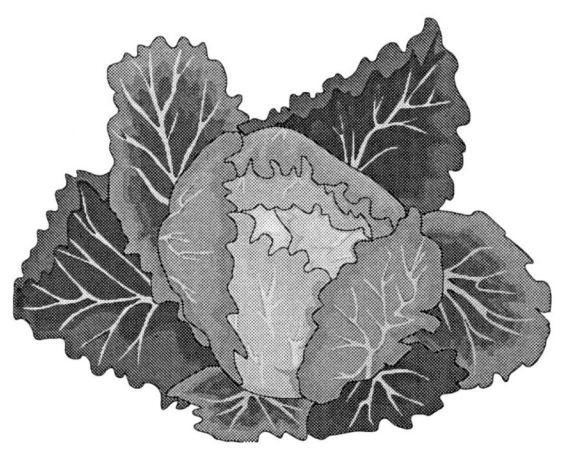

CABBAGE ROLLS II

1 medium cabbage head
1/2 cup millet
1 1/2 t. oil
1 1/2 cup water
1/2 cup grated carrots
1/2 cup onions, chopped
1 T. parsley, chopped
Mrs. Dash or Parsley Patch seasoning
1 lb. ground turkey, browned
2 cups white sauce (p. 48)

Add water to millet, cover and simmer until water is absorbed, about 30 to 35 minutes. Mix in remaining ingredients except cabbage and sauce. Cook until hot. Set aside. Steam cabbage for 10 minutes. Separate leaves and place 2 to 3 T. millet mixture into each leaf. Roll up. Put any leftover leaves and mixture in bottom of greased casserole dish. Lay rolled leaves, seam side down, in dish. Pour white sauce over all. Bake at 325 degrees for 20 minutes, covered.

SQUASH BOATS

1 acorn squash, halved lengthwise
   (or use zucchini if you have a
   tendency to fungus)
1/2 lb. ground turkey
1/2 cup chopped onion
1/2 cup chopped celery
1/2 t. thyme
dash of pepper
1 T. lemon juice
1 T. melted butter

Remove seeds and place squash in baking dish cut sides down. Add 1/2" water. Cover. Bake at 400 degrees for 15 minutes. Brown meat in a skillet; drain. Add vegetables and seasonings. Cook until vegetables are tender. Mix in lemon juice. Fill squash centers with mixture. Sprinkle butter over top. Bake uncovered 10 minutes at 400 degrees.

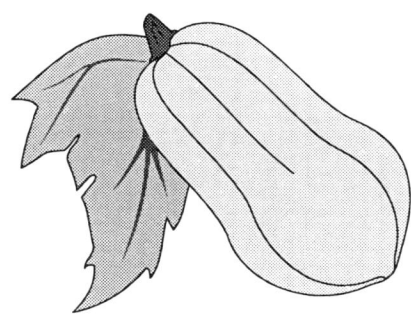

STUFFED GREEN PEPPERS

1 lb. ground turkey
1 medium onion, chopped
2 cups broth (p. 80)
1/2 cup brown rice with 2 T. wild rice
Dash of pepper
Oregano, basil, rosemary, thyme
6 green peppers

Brown meat, drain. Sauté onions in 1 T. oil. Add broth; bring to a boil. Add rice; cover and simmer until rice is tender (chewy but not soggy, about 30 minutes). Add seasonings.

Cut tops from peppers; remove core and seeds. Steam for 5 minutes. Omit precooking if a crisper texture is desired. Stuff peppers. May be frozen at this point; defrost before baking. Bake at 350 degrees for 20 minutes.

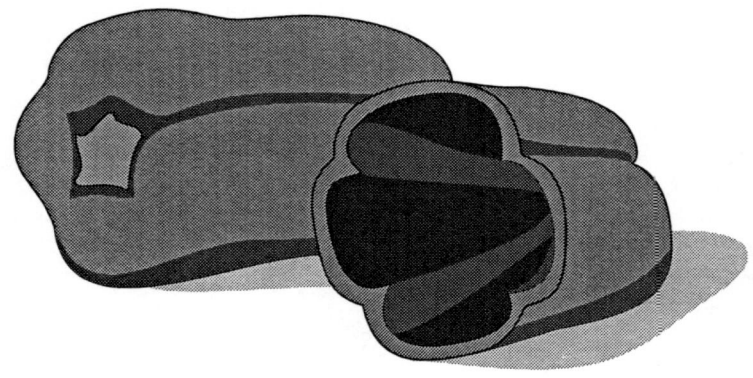

STUFFED ZUCCHINI

2 large zucchini
1 garlic clove, chopped
1 celery stalk, chopped
1/2 cup onions, chopped
1/4 cup grated carrots
1/2 cup shrimp, chopped
1/2 cup cooked brown rice

Cut zucchini in half lengthwise and steam cut side down for 5 to 7 minutes. Scoop out pulp into a large bowl and set aside. Sauté in oil or butter in a large skillet garlic, onions, celery and carrots until tender. Add shrimp and rice and cook until hot. Add to zucchini pulp and mix well. Spoon mixture back into the zucchini shells. Top with nutmeg. Broil in oven for 5 minutes.

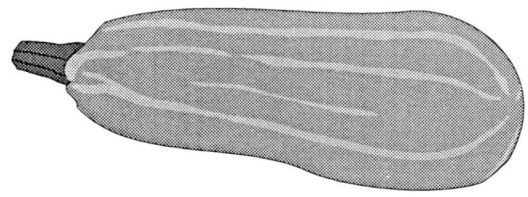

SPAGHETTI SQUASH

1/2 spaghetti squash, halved lengthwise

CLAM SAUCE:
1/4 cup olive oil
2 T. garlic cloves, chopped
2 T. oat flour or arrowroot
2 t. Italian seasonings
1/4 t. celery seed
1 can clams, drained and chopped
1 cup clam juice plus the juice from the can of clams
1 cup cooked chicken, chopped
5 to 8 cooked scallops, chopped
1 cup broccoli, steamed
1/2 cup zucchini, steamed and cubed

Steam spaghetti squash in a large skillet for 15 minutes at medium heat. While squash is steaming, prepare clam sauce.

In a saucepan, sauté garlic in olive oil. Add seasonings. Add flour or arrowroot and mix well to make a paste. Remove from heat. Slowly add clam juice and mix until smooth. Return to heat until thickened. Add clams, chicken and scallops. Set aside.

When squash is done, carefully scrape out pulp with a fork. It comes out stringy like spaghetti. Serve hot with vegetables and clam sauce poured over.

SUMMER VEGETABLE KABOBS

1 medium yellow squash
1 medium zucchini
8 small white onions
1 T. oil
5 T. cold water
3 T. lemon juice
1 1/2 t. dry mustard
1/2 t. basil
1/4 t. thyme
1/4 t. marjoram
1 small bay leaf, crumbled
1 garlic clove, minced
1 T. fresh parsley, minced
1/2 large sweet red pepper, cut into 6 equal pieces
1/2 large green pepper, cut into 6 equal pieces
    (eliminate peppers if you have arthritis)

Blanch the squash in boiling water for 5 minutes, then drain and refresh under cold running water. Blanch the zucchini and onions separately in boiling water for 7 minutes. Drain and refresh under cold running water. Cut the squash and zucchini crosswise into 16 slices each. Peel the onions.

In a large bowl combine the oil, water, lemon juice, mustard, basil, thyme, marjoram, bay leaf, garlic and parsley. Add the squash, zucchini, onions, red peppers, and green peppers to the marinade, turning carefully to coat. Cover and marinate in the refrigerator for at least 2 hours or overnight.

Remove vegetables from marinade, reserving the marinade. Arrange the vegetables on skewers. Brush with reserved marinade. Broil or grill, turning and brushing often with reserved marinade until vegetables are tender, about 10 to 12 minutes.

REFERENCE

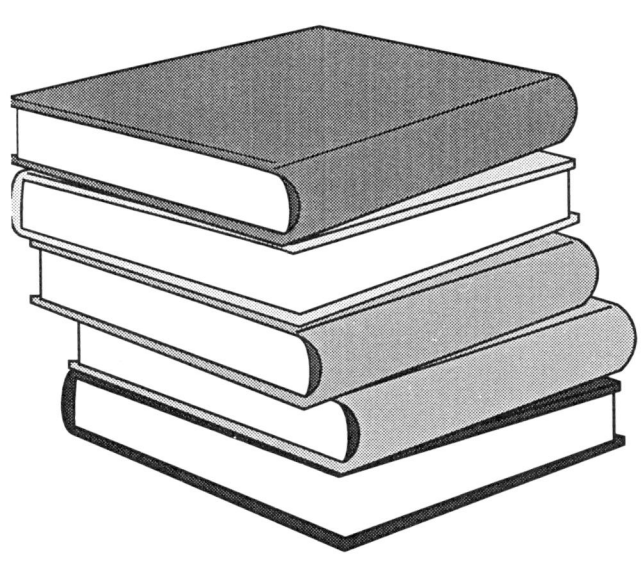

Urine Testing

Urine testing is a simple and relatively accurate way to monitor for food fermentation and overall body toxicity. It can help you find out what foods you can eat, which can change as your health changes. The pH, or relative acidity or alkalinity, of the urine can help provide this information. pH test paper is used for the testing.

Obtain pH paper, which is sold at Comprehensive Health Centers - Medical Center or at some drugstores. The pH range needed is about 4.5-7.5.

Test your urine first thing in the morning. Briefly dip a 1-2 inch strip of the pH paper into the urine stream toward the end of your first urination (if the sample is taken at the beginning of urination, sediment can give you a false pH reading). Compare the color of the wet part of the strip with the color guide on the pH paper dispenser to find out your urine pH. It is a good idea to keep a record of your diet and your urine pH on the following day to establish correlations.

Urine pH should be between 5.8 and 6.2. A reading that is higher than this can indicate fermentation of or allergy to food, and that food should be reduced or eliminated from your diet until your health and therefore your digestion improves. Some experimentation can narrow down exactly which foods are causing the problem. A reading that is too low can also indicate fermentation in a different stage - with fermentation, the pH can rise and then suddenly drop as a vinegar-like substance is made. A low reading can also indicate chemical or metal toxicity.

How urine testing relates to foods eaten:
Foods can be roughly grouped into four categories:

1. Avoid - ideally don't eat this food at all - high fungus feeding or allergenic potential.

2. Restrict - once in a while probably won't hurt you, but eat only infrequently if at all.

3. Limit - okay to eat in moderation.

4. Permitted at any time in any quantity, although food rotation may be advisable.

Any personal allergies or sensitivities, or special dietary advice from your doctor, can move a particular food to a more restrictive level.

As your health improves, you will probably be able to tolerate more foods and eat them more often without ill effect. If your urine pH stays in the normal range for five consecutive days after eating certain foods, that food can be moved up to the next level. If, for example, you have normal urine pH after eating peas or carrots, ordinarily in the Restrict category, they can be moved to the Limit category and eaten in moderation. As your health approaches an optimal level, most foods will be in the first two categories and then even a hot fudge sundae occasionally won't be a problem.

Food List

Use this chart as a rough guide to what you can eat and how much. Also be guided by your urine test results, your doctor's advice, and your own sensitivities and allergies.

The reason for not eating the food is listed next to the food., S = too sweet, A = high allergic potential, F = fungus feeder (which would also be true of anything labeled too sweet), T = toxic, R = rancid fat

Avoid (don't eat at all)

Vegetables

Beets	S
Carrot juice	S
Corn	S, A
Mushrooms	F
Sweet potatoes	S
Tomatoes	S, A

Fruits all S

Apricots
Bananas
Cherries
Citrus - Grapefruit, Oranges, Tangerines
Currants
Dates
Figs
Grapes
Peaches
Pears
Pineapple
Plums
Prunes
Raisins
Strawberries   A

Grains   A
Wheat - Wheat Flour, Bulghur wheat, Cous cous, Bread

Dairy
Milk   A
Cheese   A
Cottage cheese A

Oils
Heated oils, Fried foods   T, R
Margarine   T, R

Other
Sweets - sugar, honey, syrup, corn syrup   S
Vinegar - most mayonnaise, salad dressing, ketchup, prepared
    mustard   F
Artificial sweeteners - Saccharin, Nutri-Sweet   T
Caffeine   T, F
Alcohol   T, F

Restrict (Eat very little)
Vegetables
Carrots   S
Eggplant   A
Peppers, red   S, A

Fruit   all S
Apples
Berries - blackberries, blueberries, raspberries
Melons - cantaloupe, watermelon
Pumpkin

Beans and Legumes

Kidney beans	A, F
Lentils	A, F
Lima beans	A, F
Peas, fresh	A, F
Peas, dried	A, F
Pinto beans	A, F

Protein

Beef	T, R
Eggs (hard-cooked)	Cholesterol

Limit (eat in moderation)

Vegetables

Avocado	
Peppers, green	A
Potatoes	
Radishes	
Squash, winter	S

Beans and Legumes

Black-eyed peas
Soybeans

Fruit

Cranberries	S
Lemons, Limes	A

Grains

Barley	A
Rye	A

Triticale	A
Oat groats	A
Kamut or spelt (see p. 9)	A

Dairy
Butter
Yogurt (see p. 14)   A

Permitted

Vegetables
Artichokes
Asparagus
Beet greens
Broccoli
Brussels sprouts
Cabbage
Cauliflower
Celery
Chicory
Chives
Collard greens
Cucumbers
Dandelion greens
Endive
Escarole
Green beans
Jerusalem artichokes
Kale
Kohlrabi
Leeks
Lettuce
Mustard greens
Okra

Olives (w/o vinegar)
Onion
Parsley
Parsnips
Rhubarb
Rutabaga
Sauerkraut (w/o vinegar)
Scallions
Spinach
Squash, summer
Swiss chard
Turnip greens
Turnips
Watercress
Wax beans

Grains
Brown rice
Amaranth
Millet
Buckwheat groats
Quinoa
Teff

Protein
Fish
Lamb
Eggs (soft cooked or raw)
Chicken, Turkey

Oils
Omega I - olive oil
Omega III - salmon, mackerel, cold water fish,
    flaxseed, canola oils
Omega VI - sesame, safflower, sunflower oils

Fruits and Vegetables Classified as to Their Carbohydrate Content

The lower the carbohydrate content, the less likely the vegetable is to ferment. See discussion on fermentation, pp. 7-8.

Carbohydrate content of vegetables should also be taken into consideration when balancing carbohydrates, protein, and vegetables in a 40/30/30 ratio.

3% Vegetables

Asparagus
Bamboo shoots
Beet greens
Bean sprouts
Broccoli
Cabbage
Cauliflower
Celery
Chard
Cucumber
Lettuce
Mushrooms
Mustard greens
Parsley
Radishes
Sauerkraut
Squash, summer
Tomatoes
Turnip tops
Watercress

6% Vegetables

Beans, green
Beans, wax
Eggplant
Leeks
Parsley
Okra
Pepper, green
Pepper, red
Pumpkin
Squash, winter
Tomatoes
Turnips

6% Fruits

Cantaloupe
Honeydew
Watermelon
Strawberries

9% Vegetables
Artichokes
Beets
Brussels Sprouts
Carrots
Onions
Rutabagas

9% Fruits
Blackberries
Cranberries
Currants
Grapefruit
Lemons
Limes
Papaya
Tangerines
Gooseberries

15% Vegetables
Beans, red
Kidney beans,
  canned
Peas

15% Fruits
Apples
Blueberries
Huckleberries
Mangos
Nectarines
Pears

12% Vegetables
Soybeans, dry

12% Fruits
Cherries, sour
Loganberries
Oranges
Peaches
Pineapple
Plums
Raspberries

18% Vegetables
Horseradish
Potatoes

18% Fruits
Cherries, sweet
Crabapples
Figs, fresh
Pomegranates
Grapes

21% Vegetables
Beans, lima, fresh
Corn, fresh

21% Fruits
Banana
Prunes

Food Exchange Lists

As discussed previously, it is important to balance the food groups. The following lists tell how many servings of each food group one should have based on approximate calorie requirements. After that, permitted foods along with the amount that defines a serving are listed.

Three calorie groups are 1200, 1800, and 2400 calories a day. A woman who is trying to lose weight should follow the 1200 calorie list; a woman who isn't trying to lose weight or a man who is should follow the 1800 calorie diet, and a man who isn't trying to lose weight should follow the 2400 calorie diet.

These recommendations include the use of UltraClear protein powder (UltraBalance Inc., a division of HealthComm International Inc.). These lists are from their booklet.

If allowed (urine pH is normal for one week) fruit can be eaten. 3 servings of fruit can replace 1 protein, 1 starch, and 2 vegetables.

1200 calorie diet

6 scoops of UltraClear
3 servings protein
4 servings starch
8 servings vegetables
2 servings fat

1800 calorie diet

6 scoops of UltraClear
5 servings protein
8 servings starch
12 servings vegetables
3 servings fat

2400 calorie diet
6 scoops of UltraClear
6 servings protein
14 servings starch
12 servings vegetables
4 servings fat

Protein

Chicken, turkey	1 oz.
Dried beans	2/3 cup, cooked
Fish	1 oz.
Lamb	1 oz.
Lentils	1/2 cup cooked

Starch

Nut milk	3/4 cup
Rice	1/3 cup, cooked
Rice cakes	2
Rice milk	1/2 cup
Tapioca	2 T

Vegetables

Alfalfa sprouts	Unlimited
Artichoke	1/2 medium
Asparagus	8 spears
Bean sprouts	Unlimited
Bell peppers	1 cup raw
Broccoli	1/2 cup
Brussels sprouts	1/2 cup
Cabbage	1/2 cup cooked, 1 cup raw
Carrots	1/2 cup
Cauliflower	1/2 cup
Celery	Unlimited
Chard	1 cup
Cucumber	Unlimited
Eggplant	1/2 cup
Green or yellow beans, 1/2 cup
Jicama	1/2 cup
Kale	1/2 cup
Leeks	Unlimited
LettuceUnlimited

Mustard greens	1 cup
Okra	1/2 cup
Onions	1/2 cup cooked, 1 cup raw
Potatoes	1 small
Radishes	Unlimited
Snow peas	1/2 cup cooked
Spinach	1/2 cup cooked, 1 cup raw
Squash, summer	1/2 cup
Turnips	1/2 cup
Water chestnuts	1/2 cup
Zucchini	1 cup

Fat

Avocado	1/8
Flax oil	1 tsp.
Nuts, any type	1/2 oz.
Nut or seed butter	1 T
Oil, any type	1 tsp.
Pumpkin seeds	1/2 oz.
Sunflower seeds	1/2 oz.

Fruit, if allowed

Apples	1 small
Applesauce	1/2 cup
Apricots	2
Blueberries	3/4 cup
Kiwi	1
Melon	1 cup
Papaya	1 cup
Pears	1
Peaches	1
Pineapple	1/2 cup
Plums	2
Raspberries	1 cup

HERB AND SPICE CHART

NOTE: These are listed for your information. Foods mentioned may not necessarily be on your diet.

Seasonings can add more than flavor. Some herbs and spices also have beneficial medicinal effects:

- Ginger — Promotes sweating
- Garlic — Antimicrobial
- Cayenne — Stomach, runny nose
- Licorice — Stomach, runny nose
- Myrrh — Antifungal
- Herbal bitters — Increase HCl in stomach

HERB, SPICE OR BLEND	SUGGESTED USE:
ALLSPICE	Vegetables
BASIL	Italian dishes, soups, stews, beans, peas, and squash. Sprinkle on lamb before cooking.
BAY LEAVES	Soups and stews, fish chowder, tomato and seafood aspics. Remove before eating food.
CARAWAY	Rice or poultry.
CAYENNE PEPPER	Hot and spicy. Use in deviled eggs.

CELERY SEED	Spice mixtures, sauces, salads, salad dressings, fish and vegetables.
CHERVIL	Soups, sauces, salads and in poultry and fish stuffings.
CHILI POWDER	Good in seafood-cocktail sauces and barbecue sauces, meatloaf, hamburger and stews.
CHIVES	Salad and salad dressings, poached eggs, meat or mixed with grains.
CINNAMON	Tea and hot drinks, breakfast grains.
CLOVES	Use with cinnamon over grains.
CORIANDER	Spanish rice, Curry blends, sausage.
CRAB BOIL AND SHRIMP SPICE	Add one envelope to a quart of water when boiling shellfish.
CREAM OF TARTAR	Keeps whipped egg whites stiff.
CUMIN	Chili, hot tamales, soups, meat and rice dishes, deviled eggs, meatloaf.
CURRY POWDER	Curry sauces for eggs, vegetables, fish and meat. French dressing, clam and fish chowders and split pea soups.
DILL WEED	Soups, salads, sauces, meat and fish dishes, potatoes and potato salad, coleslaw, cucumber salad.

FENNEL	Soups, fruit dishes and sauces.
GARLIC	Most soups, salads, sauces, meats, fish and casserole dishes.
GINGER	Indian foods, pot roasts, stews, chicken, soups and fish dishes.
MACE	Fish and meat stuffings mixed with ginger. Oyster stew, poached eggs.
MARJORAM	Vegetables, lamb, sausage, stews, poultry and stuffing.
MINT	Used most often fresh in drinks, salads, fish sauces, vegetables, meat sauces (especially lamb) and soups.
MUSTARD	Cabbage, coleslaw, potato salad, soups, eggs, seafood dishes, salad dressing, meatloaf.
NUTMEG	Rice, vegetables, soups, fish dishes.
OREGANO	Almost any Italian dish, vegetable or salad.
PAPRIKA	Used as a garnish for colorless foods, fish, salads and canapés. Important ingredient in chicken paprikash and Hungarian goulash.
PARSLEY	Eggs, fish, meats, poultry, salads, sauces and vegetables.

POPPY SEED	Sprinkle over noodles, salad greens.
POULTRY SEASONING	Used to enhance the taste of poultry dishes or with paprika for meat loaf.
RED PEPPER	Spicy seasoning. Meats, sauces, fish and egg dishes.
ROSEMARY	Boiled potatoes, turnips and cauliflower. Sprinkle on chicken and fish before cooking.
SAFFRON	Adds a distinctive flavor to grains, rice and poultry.
SAGE	Poultry and soups.
SAVORY	Meats, poultry and fish dishes, poached eggs, cabbage, peas, salads.
SESAME SEED	Use in chicken dishes or sprinkled over green beans and asparagus.
TARRAGON	Chicken dishes and stuffings, green and seafood salads.
THYME	Clam sauce, fish sauces, fresh salads and egg dishes. Gives an Italian flavor to foods.
TURMERIC	Add to dressing.

INDEX

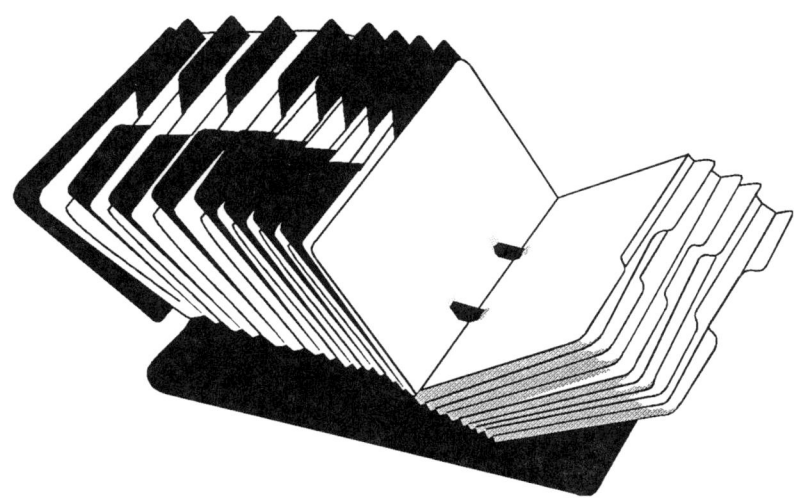

INDEX

Gravies
Basic White Sauce   48
Brown Gravy   49

Hot Cereal
Roasted Grain Breakfast Cream Cereal   30

Marinade
Marinade I - For Fish   57
Marinade II - For Chicken   57

Mayonnaise
Curried Mayonnaise Dressing   50
Mayonnaise   47
Mustard-Mayonnaise Sauce   52

Meatballs
Icelandic Meatballs   135
Lemon-Parsley Meatballs   136
Russian Minted Meatballs   38

Millet
Millet and Vegetables   149
Millet Croquettes   96
Millet Muffins   27

Muffins
Millet Muffins   27
Salmon Muffins   41
Tuna Muffins   42
Veggie Muffins   42

Mustard
Mustard   58
Zucchini Mustard   51

Mariner's Salad	72
Minnesota Chicken Salad	74
Potato Salad	67
Potato and Egg Salad	62
Quinoa-Vidalia Salad	73
Rice Salad	64
Tabouli Salad	73
Tossed Green Salad	61
Veggie-Potato Salad	62
Yogurt Salad	66

Salmon
Salmon Muffins	41
Salmon Patties	39
Salmon Patties with Poached Egg	33
Salmon Steaks with Curried Avocado Sauce	145
Steamed Eggs with Salmon	27

Sauces
Basic White Sauce	48
Brown Gravy	49
Cashew Sauce	52
Classic Hollandaise Sauce	55
Creamy Dill Sauce	57
Curry Sauce	51
Curry Sauce with Nuts	51
Dilled Cucumber Sauce	53
Lemon-Butter Sauce	56
Mild Indian Sauce	52
Mustard-Mayonnaise Sauce	52
Peggy's Pesto	58

Sausage
Easy Breakfast Sausage	25
Italian Sausage	25